Zone Cooking Made Easy

6 Weeks of Delicious
Zone Balanced Meals

by
Faye Hoffoss

© 2002 by Faye Hoffoss. All rights reserved.

No part of this book may be reproduced, stored in a retrieval system, or transmitted by any means, electronic, mechanical, photocopying, recording, or otherwise, without written permission from the author.

ISBN: 0-7596-6670-9

This book is printed on acid free paper.

Dedication

This book is dedicated to my daughter, Diane. Not only has she been my inspiration, but has been there for me every step of the way. No matter how busy, she found the time to listen and give advice. And, thanks to her, I have found the courage to write my own cookbook.

Useful Information

Extra Virgin Olive Oil: People that use extra virgin olive oil in place of vegetable or Canola oil have better cholesterol and blood pressure; have less heart disease, cancer and arthritis; and tend to live longer. New research shows that diets rich in extra virgin olive oil even help prevent wrinkles.

Whole Grains: Eating whole grains can reduce your odds of heart disease, cancer, diabetes, obesity and premature death. (Examples: oatmeal, shredded wheat, whole grain bread, brown rice, and popcorn.) Whole grains deliver lots of fiber, antioxidants, anti-cancer agents, cholesterol reducers, clot blockers, and essential minerals.

Fatty Fish: Fresh or canned salmon, tuna, sardines and mackerel boosts health. These are the only fish to have lots of omega-3 oils to keep arteries clear, hearts in rhythm, and the brain and joints functioning well. Eating fatty fish once a week decreases your risk of a fatal heart attack by 44%.

Tea: Brewed tea (from bags or loose tea) has an amazing power to help discourage stroke, heart attack, cancer and neurological damage. Although black and green tea are about equal in overall antioxidant protection, the green tea has EGCG, a unique anti-cancer agent and brain cell protector. Brew the tea five minutes. Instant, bottled and herbal teas don't work as they lack antioxidants.

Fruit and Vegetables: Plant foods are the best antidote to virtually all chronic ailments: high blood pressure, heart disease, diabetes, cancer, arthritis, stroke, wrinkles, obesity, and age-related mental decline. Fruits and vegetables are rich in vitamins, minerals, fiber and antioxidants. Berries, citrus fruits and dark green vegetables are best. Eat at least 5 servings a day.

Low Glycemic Carbohydrates: High glycemic carbohydrates spike blood sugar and insulin. Low glycemic carbohydrates do not. Low insulin contributes to longevity. Eating low glycemic carbohydrates such as, dried beans, lentils, peanuts, yogurt, oatmeal, cherries, and prunes can help prevent colon cancer, heart disease, diabetes, weight gain and poor memory.

Meat, Animal Fat, Trans Fat and Salt: All can wreck your body. Red meat, (especially fried, as bacon), is linked to colon cancer, so it's best to eat in small portions, (3 to 4 oz) Saturated fat in whole milk, butter cheese, sausage, steak and poultry clogs arteries; as do Trans fatty acids in many margarines, processed snacks and baked goods. (Partially hydrogenated found on a food label indicates Trans fats.) Excess salt can shorten your life and bring on heart disease even if your blood pressure is good.

Eat Less: By cutting your portion size you can do more to improve your health than anything else you may do. The harder your body has to work to process excess calories the more you speed up aging, cancer, heart disease, diabetes and Alzheimer's disease. Trimming calories along with any mild, regular exercise is the only reliable way known to increase your life span.

Vitamins: A lack of micro-nutrients such as folic acid, niacin, zinc and vitamins B12, B6, C and E, damages DNA the same way radiation and chemicals do, setting the stage for cancer. Correcting even minor deficiencies can boost immunity, curb chronic diseases and perhaps prolong your life.

Foreword

I should begin by saying that I do not have a formal education in nutrition. I am a wife and mother who has worked for years, trying to keep my family fit and healthy. We have tried several different diets over the years, but none of them had lasting success until we found "The Zone" diet.

My daughter, Diane, introduced me to a couple of books written by Dr. Barry Sears.
The first, "The Zone," I found very hard to understand. His next book, "Mastering The Zone," was a little easier to read, but still very hard to put into practice. I don't know exactly why this diet works so well, but when we stay in "The Zone," the fat melts away. "The Zone" diet is based on eating meals in which the PCF's (proteins, carbohydrates, and fats) are "balanced". This maximizes the body's fat burning characteristics. The problem with this diet is that it requires a lot of math. You have to calculate the blocks of PCF's in a recipe, make adjustments and then recalculate. You do this over and over until the meal is properly balanced. Diane didn't have a problem with this, but then she has a Ph.D. in mathematics.

I went to the bookstore to try to find a book that had meals that were already balanced. When I did find one, it used a lot of "diet foods." I knew from experience that my family would not stay with this diet if they had to eat tofu, alfalfa sprouts, watercress, protein powder, soy products, and etc. They wanted to be able to eat the way we normally ate, and still lose weight. At that time I thought it would be an impossible task.

Back to the bookstore again; determined to find a cookbook with recipes we could live with. None! I was ready to give up, but my daughter wouldn't let me. She found one called "40-30-30 Fat Burning Nutrition," by Joyce and Gene Daoust. Their book made more sense, but again, although the foods were closer to the way we were eating, they were still just too different.

With Diane's encouragement, I started trying to adapt my everyday meals to "The Zone." It was a slow and tedious process, but I kept at it. The result was almost unbelievable: my family didn't even know they were on a diet most of the time. Other family members and friends began asking about our weight loss, and I recommended the above Zone diet books to them. They all complained that the book was too hard to understand, weren't crazy about some of the "diet foods," and the math too difficult.
When they tried some of my pre-balanced recipes, they loved them. They found the diet easy to stick with as long as they didn't have to go through all the math calculations.

I think "The Zone" diet is wonderful. By eating this way, not only have I lost weight, but I have been able to sleep through the night and awaken in the morning virtually pain free. This in itself was wonderful, but I soon found many other great side effects. I now feel more alert, and have more energy. I no longer have gas or bloating, my heartburn is gone, I feel happier, my clothes fit better and the pounds just keep melting away. Food is no longer on my mind every waking moment, and I am never hungry.

My husband had been sleeping with his head on 3 or 4 pillows to combat his heartburn, but now he sleeps with just one. Our blood pressure and cholesterol levels are in a very acceptable zone. This was all the extra encouragement I needed. I became a zealot. I told everyone I knew about "The Zone." (And even people I didn't know.)

I adapted more and more of my recipes to Zone meals, and tried each one out on my family. The meals they gave me the thumbs up on were added to this book. Believe me, it wasn't easy. I drove my daughter crazy with all my questions, expecting her to know the answers. After all, not only is she a math professor, but she had two friends on "The Zone," and they were losing weight. (It was amazing how much they had lost.)

I am sure there were days when my family wanted to run away from home. (I know I did.) Instead, each time I attempted to balance a new meal, they would make suggestions on how I could make it taste better. Next I started on my friends and other family members. I sent them sample recipes to try out and got feedback from them as well.

What follows are some hints and ideas that made it easier for us to stay on this diet. "Diet?" It's not really a diet, just a way to fix meals that are balanced, healthier, and easier on the taste buds.

I have no idea what Dr. Barry Sears or Joyce and Gene Daoust would say about my meals, but it is working for us. I have found meals that my family will eat and still lose weight. Hopefully, as time goes by I will learn more about the process and make my recipes better and healthier. But for now, not only does my family no longer frown at me over the dinner table, they are also healthier and more fit. What more could a mother ask!

Library of Congress Cataloging in Publication
Faye C. Hoffoss
Includes index.
TXu 907-907   June 7, 1999
Zone Cooking Made Easy

Table of Contents

	Page
Useful Information	v
Foreword	vii
6-Week Daily Menu Plan	xi
Introduction	xvii
What is a Block?	1
Finding Your Daily Block Size	2
Helpful Hints	3
Staying Balanced When Traveling:	6
Eating in Restaurants: Breakfast Examples:	7
Lunch Examples	7
Dinner Examples	8
Eating at Fast Food Restaurants: Lunches or Dinners:	10
6 weeks of planned meals.	11
Beginning Weight and Measurements	12
Staples Shopping List	13
Week 1 - Grocery List	14
Week 1 - Planned Meals	15
Week 1 - Results	30
Week 2 - Grocery List	31
Week 2 - Planned Meals	33
Week 2 - Results	48
Week 3 - Grocery List	49
Week 3 - Planned Meals	50
Week 3 - Results	66
Week 4 - Grocery List	67
Week 4 - Planned Meals	68
Week 4 - Results	84
Week 5 - Grocery List	85
Week 5 - Planned Meals	86
Week 5 - Results	102
Week 6 - Grocery List	103

- Week 6 - Planned Meals ---104
- Week 6 - 12 Results ---120
- Alternative Meals ---127
  - Breakfast Choices ---128
  - Lunch Choices ---145
  - Beef Dinner Choices ---157
  - Chicken Dinner Choices ---181
  - Fish Dinner Choices ---212
  - Pork Dinner Choices ---232
  - Vegetarian Dinner Choices ---240
- 2 Block Snack Choices ---245
- Holiday Meals Section ---251
- Miscellaneous Choices ---254
  - Honey Wheat Bread ---255
  - Unbalanced Salads ---256
  - Salad DressingsMarinades and Sauces ---257
- Balanced 3-Block Salads ---260
- Food Guide Section ---268
- Index ---286
- References ---293

6-Week Daily Menu Plan

Week 1:	Breakfasts	Page #	Block #
Day 1:	Eggs with Ham and Orange Juice	16	3
Day 2:	Eggs Benedict	18	3
Day 3:	Eggs and Grapefruit	20	3
Day 4:	Malt-O-Meal	22	4
Day 5:	Wheaties	24	3
Day 6:	Eggs with Cheese and Bacon	26	3
Day 7:	French Toast with Sausage	28	4

Week 1:	Lunches	Page #	Block #
Day 1:	Ham and Cheese Sandwich with Grapes	16	3
Day 2:	Tuna Melt	18	2
Day 3:	Roast Beef Sandwich	20	3
Day 4:	Bacon, Lettuce and Tomato Sandwich with Cheese	22	3
Day 5:	Hot Ham and Swiss Sandwich	24	2
Day 6:	Hot Pastrami	26	3
Day 7:	Beef with Vegetable and Barley Soup	28	2

Eat a 1-Block Snack between Lunch and Dinner every day.
2-Block Snacks can be found on Pages 246 - 250.
Divide the 2-Block Snack in half and save the other half for later.

Week 1:	Dinners	Page #	Block #
Day 1:	Steak and French Fries for 3	17	4
Day 2:	Chicken Cutlet Parmesan for 3	19	5
Day 3:	Salmon Patties for 3	21	5
Day 4:	Chicken a la Marengo for 3	23	4
Day 5:	Pork Teriyaki with Orange Salad for 3	25	4
Day 6:	Texas Hash for 4	27	4
Day 7:	Chicken Breasts with Sour Cherry Sauce for 3	29	4

Eat a 1-Block Snack about 1/2 Hour before bed every day.
2-Block Snacks can be found on Pages 246 - 250.
Divide the 2-Block Snack in half and save the other half for later.

6-Week Daily Menu Plan

Week 2:	Breakfasts	Page #	Block #
Day 1:	Eggs with Ham and Orange Juice	34	3
Day 2:	Sausage and Eggs with Cantaloupe	36	3
Day 3:	Omelet with Ham and Orange Juice	38	4
Day 4:	Smart Start	40	3
Day 5:	Eggs with Ham and Cheese	42	3
Day 6:	Oatmeal	44	3
Day 7:	French Toast with Ham	46	3

Week 2:	Lunches	Page #	Block #
Day 1:	Tuna Sandwich	35	3
Day 2:	Vegetarian Vegetable Soup and Ham Sandwich	37	3
Day 3:	Grilled Ham and Cheese Sandwich	39	2
Day 4:	Hot Ham and Swiss Sandwich	44	3
Day 5:	Egg Salad Sandwich	43	2
Day 6:	Tuna Melt	45	3
Day 7:	Hot Ham and Swiss	47	3

Eat a 1-Block Snack between Lunch and Dinner every day.
2-Block Snacks can be found on Pages 246 - 250.
Divide the 2-Block Snack in half and save the other half for later.

Week 2:	Dinners	Page #	Block #
Day 1:	Grilled Orange Roughy and Apple Cole Slaw for 3	35	4
Day 2:	Steak and Potatoes for 3	37	4
Day 3:	Garlic Chicken with Angel Food Cake for 3	39	4
Day 4:	Cheesy Orange Roughy for 3	41	4
Day 5:	Pork Roast and Vegetables for 3	43	5
Day 6:	Lasagna for 6	45	5
Day 7:	Chicken Cacciatore for 3	47	4

Eat a 1-Block Snack about 1/2 Hour before bed every day.
2-Block Snacks can be found on Pages 246 -250.
Divide the 2-Block Snack in half and save the other half for later.

6-Week Daily Menu Plan

Week 3:	**Breakfasts**	Page #	Block #
Day 1:	Eggs with Ham and Salsa	52	3
Day 2:	Oatmeal with Ham and Cheese	54	3
Day 3:	Eggs Benedict	56	3
Day 4:	French Toast with Ham	58	3
Day 5:	Omelet with Ham and Cheese	60	3
Day 6:	Poached Eggs with English Toasting Bread	62	2
Day 7:	French Toast with Ham	64	4

Week 3:	**Lunches**	Page #	Block #
Day 1:	Ham and American Cheese Sandwich with Grapes	52	3
Day 2:	Tuna Melt	54	2
Day 3:	Beef with Vegetable and Barley and Tuna Sandwich	56	3
Day 4:	Roast Beef Sandwich	58	3
Day 5:	Tuna Sandwich	60	3
Day 6:	Ham and Swiss Cheese Sandwich with Grapes	62	3
Day 7:	Grilled Ham and Cheese Sandwich	64	2

Eat a 1-Block Snack between Lunch and Dinner every day.
2-Block Snacks can be found on Pages 246 - 250.
Divide the 2-Block Snack in half and save the other half for later.

Week 3:	**Dinners**	Page #	Block #
Day 1:	Shrimp Scampi for 3	53	4
Day 2:	Beef Bourguignon for 3	55	5
Day 3:	Teriyaki Chicken with Fruit Salad for 3	57	4
Day 4:	Cheesy Fillet of Sole for 3	59	4
Day 5:	Pork Loin Chops with Cole Slaw for 3	61	4
Day 6:	Beef Stroganoff for 3	63	5
Day 7:	Chicken and Stuffing Bake for 3	65	4

Eat a 1-Block Snack about 1/2 Hour before bed every day.
2-Block Snacks can be found on Pages 246 - 250.
Divide the 2-Block Snack in half and save the other half for later.

6-Week Daily Menu Plan

Week 4:	Breakfasts	Page #	Block #
Day 1:	Sausage and Eggs with Orange Juice	70	3
Day 2:	Eggs with Toast and ham	72	4
Day 3:	Sausage & Eggs with Potatoes and Strawberries	74	3
Day 4:	Shredded Wheat	76	2
Day 5:	Omelet with Ham and Cheese	78	3
Day 6:	Sausage and Eggs with Potatoes and Jam	80	3
Day 7:	French Toast with Ham	82	3

Week 4:	Lunches	Page #	Block #
Day 1:	Tuna Sandwich	70	3
Day 2:	Beef with Vegetable and Barley Soup	72	2
Day 3:	Hot Pastrami	74	3
Day 4:	Reuben Sandwich	76	4
Day 5:	Ham and Swiss Cheese Sandwich	78	3
Day 6:	Tuna Melt	80	3
Day 7:	Chicken Noodle Soup and Ham Sandwich	82	3

Eat a 1-Block Snack between Lunch and Dinner every day.
2-Block Snacks can be found on Pages 246 - 250.
Divide the 2-Block Snack in half and save the other half for later.

Week 4:	Dinners	Page #	Block #
Day 1:	Grilled Halibut for 3	71	4
Day 2:	Meat Loaf for 3	73	4
Day 3:	Orange Chicken with Green Grapes for 3	75	4
Day 4:	Stuffed Orange Roughy for 3	77	4
Day 5:	Pork Chops with Stuffing for 3	79	4
Day 6:	Spaghetti for 6	81	4
Day 7:	Chicken Dijon with Ginger Pear Sauce for 3	83	4

Eat a 1-Block Snack about 1/2 Hour before bed every day.
2-Block Snacks can be found on Pages 246 - 250.
Divide the 2-Block Snack in half and save the other half for later.

6-Week Daily Menu Plan

Week 5:	**Breakfasts**	**Page #**	**Block #**
Day 1:	Shredded Wheat	88	3
Day 2:	Ham and Eggs with Cheese and Grapefruit	90	3
Day 3:	French Toast with Ham	92	3
Day 4:	Eggs with Toast and Jam	94	3
Day 5:	Eggs Benedict	96	3
Day 6:	Sausage and Eggs with Potatoes and Jam	98	3
Day 7:	Poached Egg with English Toasting Bread	100	2

Week 5:	**Lunches**	**Page #**	**Block #**
Day 1:	Tuna Sandwich	88	3
Day 2:	Roast Beef Sandwich	90	3
Day 3:	Toasted Tomato Sandwich and 2% Cottage Cheese	92	3
Day 4:	Grilled Ham and Cheese Sandwich	94	3
Day 5:	Vegetarian Vegetable Soup and Ham Sandwich	96	3
Day 6:	Ham and American Cheese Sandwich with Grapes	98	3
Day 7:	Tuna Melt	100	3

Eat a 1-Block Snack between Lunch and Dinner every day.
2-Block Snacks can be found on Pages 246 - 250.
Divide the 2-Block Snack in half and save the other half for later.

Week 5:	**Dinners**	**Page #**	**Block #**
Day 1:	Fillet of Sole for 3	89	4
Day 2:	Chicken with Orange Peel Szechwan Style for 3	91	4
Day 3:	Beef Stew for 6	93	4
Day 4:	Chicken Drumsticks with Angel Food Cake for 3	95	5
Day 5:	Veal with Vegetable and Gravy for 3	97	4
Day 6:	Fish and Chips for 3	99	4
Day 7:	Chicken Cordon Bleu	101	5

Eat a 1-Block Snack about 1/2 Hour before bed every day.
2-Block Snacks can be found on Pages 246 - 250.
Divide the 2-Block Snack in half and save the other half for later.

6-Week Daily Menu Plan

Week 6:	**Breakfasts**	Page #	Block #
Day 1:	Eggs with Ham and Cheese	102	3
Day 2:	Poached Eggs with English Toasting Bread	104	2
Day 3:	Smart Start	106	3
Day 4:	Eggs and Grapefruit	108	2
Day 5:	Breakfast Tortilla	110	3
Day 6:	Special K	112	3
Day 7:	Ham and Eggs with Grapefruit	114	3

Week 6:	**Lunches**	Page #	Block #
Day 1:	Tuna Sandwich	102	3
Day 2:	Reuben Sandwich	104	4
Day 3:	Hot Ham and Swiss Sandwich	106	3
Day 4:	Ham and Swiss Sandwich with Grapes (1 1/2 Sandwiches)	108	4
Day 5:	Grilled Ham and Cheese Sandwich	110	2
Day 6:	Chicken Noodle Soup and Ham Sandwich	112	3
Day 7:	Bacon Lettuce and Tomato with Cheese	114	3

Eat a 1-Block Snack between Lunch and Dinner every day.
2-Block Snacks can be found on Pages 246 - 250.
Divide the 2-Block Snack in half and save the other half for the later.

Week 6:	**Dinners**	Page #	Block #
Day 1:	Chicken with Peach Sauté for 3	103	4
Day 2:	Boneless B.B.Q. Pork "Ribs" for 3	105	4
Day 3:	Hawaiian Chicken for 3	107	4
Day 4:	Oriental Stir-Fry Shrimp for 3	109	4
Day 5:	Bottom Round Roast with Vegetables for 3	111	5
Day 6:	Manhattan Chicken for 3	113	4
Day 7:	Steak and Fries for 3	115	4

Eat a 1-Block Snack about 1/2 Hour before bed every day.
2-Block Snacks can be found on Pages 246 - 250.
Divide the 2-Block Snack in half and save the other half for later.

Introduction
This book contains several sections:

1. A section to help you calculate the number of blocks you should be eating each day, according to your weight and activity level.

2. Hints on adapting to this new way of eating.

3. Dining out and Staying Balanced.

4. Tables to help you keep track of results.

5. A 6-week menu of planned balanced meals, providing a total of 12 blocks per day.

6. A weekly shopping lists for all the meals on the 6-week menu plan.

7. A selection of balanced breakfasts, lunches, dinners, and snacks to change a planned meal as needed. The dinners are arranged in beef, chicken, fish, pork, and vegetarian.

8. Some blocked salads you can use for lunches or dinners.

9. A Food Guide to help you adapt your own recipes.

10. An index to make it easier to find specific meals.

11. The Blocked Meals have numbers for exchanging foods in a planned meal.

12. The whole 6-Week Daily Menu Plan at a glance.

You can follow my 6-week menu plan exactly, make fruit and vegetable changes, or mix and match the meals from the alternative meals section. (Just make sure the meal you substitute contains the same number of blocks). Once you have become more comfortable cooking this way, you can start to adapt your own meals with the Food Guide section.

I made the 6-week menu section 12 block days, because that seems to be the number of blocks most people need. If you need more than 12 blocks, there are several ways you can do it: adjust the meal portions I have provided, substitute a larger block meal from the Alternative Meals section, or have larger block snacks.

I believe that if you follow the recipes in this book you will be healthier, feel better, and lose weight. Keep at it. It took me many weeks to grasp the concept and develop the ability to adapt my recipes, but now I am starting to feel almost as comfortable cooking this way as I did cooking the old way.

What is a Block?

7 grams of proteins equals **1 block** of protein.
9 grams of carbohydrates equals **1 block** of carbohydrates.
3 grams of fats equals **1 block** of fat.

1 block of protein, **plus**
1 block of carbohydrates, **plus**
1 block of fat = a **1 Block Balanced Meal**.

To balance a meal, start with the amount of protein grams on the food package label. Divide the total number of protein grams by 7. This gives you the number of "Protein Blocks." Find the number of carbohydrates grams, subtract the dietary fiber and then divide the total number of carbohydrate grams by 9. This gives you the number of "Carbohydrate Blocks." Then find the number of fat grams; divide the total number of fat grams by 3. This gives you the number of "Fat Blocks."

Add or subtract food grams to make the meal balance. (Protein Blocks, Carbohydrate Blocks, and Fat Blocks should be the same number of blocks.) It doesn't have to be exactly equal it just needs to be close.

Most people don't eat enough fiber each day, increasing their risk of colon cancer and heart disease. By adding strawberries grapes, mandarin oranges, etc in your salad, or as a dessert, not only are you eating lighter you are also consuming a little more fiber each day.

Example:
A 3 Block Zone Balanced Meal:
3 Blocks of Protein, 3 Blocks of Carbohydrates, and 3 Blocks of Fat.

If you start with a recipe or meal that has 3 blocks of protein (21 grams), 2 blocks of carbohydrates (18 grams), and 3 blocks of fat (9 grams), you should add 1 block of carbohydrates (5 to 9 grams) to make it 3 blocks.

Below is an example of one of the zone balanced 3 block meals in this book. After eating this 3-block meal, you would still have 9 blocks for the rest of the day, if you are suppose to be eating 12 blocks a day. As you can see, this meal is not exactly 3 blocks of PCF's, but it is close enough.

		P	C	F
1	Egg, Whole	6.0	0	5.0
1	Egg White	4.0	0	0
2 slice	Wheat Bread, Pepperidge Farm, light	4.0	14.0	0.5
3 slices	Honey Ham, 97% lean	5.0	1.0	0.7
2 T	Pace Salsa	0	3.0	0
4 oz.	Orange Juice	0.8	13.0	0
1 t	Butter	0	0	3.6
	Total grams	19.8	31.0	9.8
	Total blocks	2.8	3.4	3.2

Finding Your Daily Block Size

Look at the chart below. The number of blocks you will need depends on your weight and activity level.

Activity Level Hours each Week	Low to Medium 0 to 4 hours	Medium to High 5 to 10 hours
Less than 140 lbs.	11 Blocks	12 Blocks
141 - 180 lbs.	12 Blocks	13 Blocks
181 - 250+ lbs.	13 Blocks	14 Blocks

The number of blocks you start with is the number you should be eating for the rest of your life, unless your exercise level changes. You start out eating the number of blocks needed as though you were already at the ideal weight for your body.

Something I have found, and have had to learned to accept: although I would like to be a 5' 9" young woman, and as thin as a reed, I am only 5' 1", middle aged, and don't have the genetics necessary to be skinny. I have since taken a more realistic view of the facts. Now, after losing my excess weight from eating balanced meals, I find I am very happy with the results.

NOTE:

**For more information, read, "The Zone" and "Mastering The Zone" by Barry Sears, Ph.D., and/or "40-30-30 Fat Burning Nutrition," by Joyce and Gene Daoust.
They are experts in this field.**

Abbreviations used in this book
T   Tablespoon
t   Teaspoon
C   Cup
oz   Ounces

Helpful Hints

1. When I mention **PCF's** in this book, I'm talking about grams of Proteins, Carbohydrates and Fats.

2. Learn to read food labels in terms of **"Food Blocks,"** and make the necessary adjustments when you make a meal.

3. Drink a glass of water as soon as possible each morning.

4. Eat a Balanced meal within 1 hour of waking each morning.

5. Eat 3 Balanced meals and 2 Balanced snacks every day. (Don't skip any meals or snacks, as it could slow your weight loss.)

6. Eat 2 Balanced snacks a day, the first after lunch, the second, about thirty minutes before going to bed. (If you need only 1 block for each snack, you can cut any 2-block snack in half.)

7. Drink six to eight, 8 ounce glasses of water a day. (I learned to drink enough water by carrying a small bottle around with me all day.)

8. Don't skip meals. (It stops the fat burning process, you lose weight slower, and you are more likely to overeat at your next meal.) When I find myself rushed for time I will eat a 40-30-30 Balanced 2 Block Bar instead of a regular breakfast or lunch.

9. If you make a mistake, or want to eat a meal that is "not balanced," don't give up, your next "balanced meal or snack" will get you in balance again. (Don't do it very often though, you won't lose any weight, and you could start gaining.)

10. Exercise. No one in my family likes exercise programs, but we love to walk together. Walking not only helps us physically, but without the usual distractions, we find that we communicate much more. Have a 1 or 2 block balanced snack 30 minutes before walking or exercising.

11. If you want to drink an alcoholic beverage that has carbohydrates, drink it with a meal. Remember to add the carbohydrates in the drink to the carbohydrates in your meal.

12. Limit carbohydrates with high (H), medium high (M/H) or very high (V/H) Glycemic Rating (G/R). (Such as; breads, pastas, sugars, potatoes, carrots, corn, and grains.) I have Glycemic Ratings in the Food Guide under the G/R column.

13. If you are not hungry or sleepy 2 to 3 hours after your meal, your meal was properly balanced.

14. If you are hungry and sleepy, 2 to 3 hours after your meal, you've had too many carbohydrates for the number of proteins and fats. The meal is not balanced. Make the same meal next time, but decrease the carbohydrates by about 1 block.

15. If you're hungry, but not sleepy, add about 1 block of carbohydrates to the same meal next time.

16. If you drink coffee, switch to decaf or mix them in equal portions. But do it gradually to avoid withdrawals, although I am finding I don't want much coffee when on the zone.

17. Most of your carbohydrates should come from low glycemic fruits and vegetables, so use bread, starch, pasta, sugar, potatoes, corn, carrots, and grain sparingly.

18. Keep some balanced snack foods handy. (My family will just grab anything if I don't have a supply ready.) Try the Beef or Chicken Chimichangas recipe on page 248.

19. Keep all that "delicious junk food" out of the house. The temptation might be too strong.

20. Commercially prepared foods are usually too high in carbohydrates. Add some low-fat protein, like 2% cottage cheese, turkey, fish, tuna, or chicken.

21. If the commercially prepared foods are too high in protein, eat a small salad with 1 or 2 tablespoon of salad dressing, or some fresh fruit. (Or don't eat all of the protein.)

22. Most grilled or roasted chicken sandwiches without cheese will be balanced.

23. Never let more than 5 hours go by without eating a balanced meal or snack.

24. Measure carefully, it doesn't take much to make a meal unbalanced.

25. Drink an 8-ounce glass of water about 30 minutes before eating.

26. When eating a meal, eat a few bites of protein first.

27. During the first 2 or 3 weeks, try not to eat many unfavorable carbohydrates: (high-glycemic) Pasta, Bread, Rice, Potatoes, Carrots, Corn, Grains, etc.

28. Don't eat on the run. Sit down, relax, and chew your food thoroughly before swallowing.

29. Never eat less than 8 blocks of protein a day.

30. Try not to eat more than 5 Blocks per meal, 4 would be better.

31. You can drink a glass of wine with any meal. (Make sure it does not have any carbohydrates.)

32. If you can't find some of the foods with the same PCF count mentioned in this book, find one that's as close as possible in PCF's. (I have given name brands as often as possible to make it easier to find the right PCF's for each meal.)

33. Get a friend or family member to diet and exercise with you. (You can encourage and motivate each other when you get discouraged.)

34. Have fun. Find a variety of exercises that you really enjoy.

35. Be realistic. Don't compare your weight loss and fitness level with anyone else. Not everyone loses weight at the same rate.

36. Work toward a long-term goal. To make fitness a part of your life, use the weekly planner at the end of each week to keep track of your accomplishments.

37. Don't go grocery shopping when you are hungry. Use the weekly shopping list to buy your groceries. It's handy, and helps keep you from buying things you don't need.

38. Try my 6 week balanced meals and you will see fantastic results.

39. The number of protein blocks should equal the number of carbohydrate and fat blocks. Example: A"3 Block" meal consists of: 3 Blocks of Protein, 3 Blocks of Carbohydrates, and 3 Blocks of Fat. (21 grams of protein = 3 block of protein. 27 grams of carbohydrates =3 block of carbohydrates, and 9 grams of fat = 3 block of fat.)

40. It's probably a good idea to discuss this diet with your doctor. Additional vitamins, calcium, etc. may be advisable for your particular needs.

41. Remember, when cooking food for more than one person; always weigh each food item before serving to make sure you have divided properly. Don't worry, it won't be long before you will be able to divide evenly just by looking.

42. Most packaged meats aren't the exact amount needed for each recipe. After grocery shopping, I take the time to trim, weigh, package, and label the meats for each recipe before freezing. It takes a little more time, but I find the convenience at mealtime well worth the investment.

43. When making recipes larger than needed for one person per meal, divide and freeze the extra meal or meals in individual portions. You can microwave them later when you are tired or short on time; or take them to work for lunch. Then you won't be so tempted to skip a meal or grab something from a fast food place.

44. Most people only eat about half the recommended daily requirement of fiber each day, increasing their risk of colon cancer and heart disease. By adding strawberries, grapes, etc to the your meals, not only are you eating lighter you are also consuming a little more fiber each day.

45. You can substitute any fruit and/or vegetable given in the planned meals as long as the substitution has about the same PCF's as in the recipe. At times you may even omit part of the fruits and/or vegetables in the recipes and still have a balanced meal.

46. G/R stands for Glycemic Rating. The Glycemic Rating rates how fast certain foods increase blood sugar levels, and how long it takes for you body to bring it back to normal. The lower the Glycemic Rating numbers for the carbohydrates, the better your chances of losing weight faster, as they usually have more fiber, minerals and vitamins.

47. Most of the meals in this book take no more than 10 or 15 minutes preparation time.

48. I have added the name brands of many foods to make it easier to find the right balance when shopping.

Staying Balanced When Traveling:

1. Choose a low-fat protein from the menu, like grilled fish, chicken or turkey, and build your meal around it. (Order grilled or broiled meat whenever possible. Remove any skin and fat before eating.)

2. Order a la carte. That way you can choose what you eat.

3. Don't eat the rolls or chips.

4. If you really want dessert, skip all carbohydrates, (both high-glycemic, and low-glycemic) and order any dessert you want, but just eat half of it. Fresh fruit is better for you than dessert, but everyone wants to eat something sweet once in a while.

5. Ask to have the rice, potatoes, or pasta replaced with low-glycemic vegetables, or limit the high-glycemic vegetables or pasta. High-glycemic vegetables and pasta are at least twice the amount of carbohydrates as the same portion of low-glycemic vegetables.

6. When your dinner arrives, check the size of the protein. Eat only the portion that looks like it would fit in the palm of your hand. (And about the same thickness as your hand.) (It will weigh between 3 and 4 ounces.) If the carbohydrates are unfavorable, (corn, rice, potatoes, carrots, pasta, and grains) eat only half the portion. (Or half the total volume of the protein you will be eating.) If the carbohydrates are favorable, the total volume of carbohydrates should be about double the volume of the protein you will be eating.

7. Drink a glass of wine instead of snacking on appetizers. If you have an appetizer, make it high protein. (Shrimp, Salmon, or Chicken.)

8. Get a room with a microwave and go to a supermarket. There are several well-known brands of healthy, low-fat frozen dinners available today. Not all of the meals are balanced but many of them are. Most seem to be about 3 blocks (21g of protein, 27g of carbohydrates, and 9g of fat).

9. Avoid beverages that contain sugar.

10. Some restaurant water tastes better if you add a lemon wedge.

11. Avoid fried foods when eating out; and when frying foods at home, use non-fat spray with oil or butter sparingly.

12. Eat a 1 or 2 block snack before bedtime. (It keeps your body working while you sleep.)

Eating in Restaurants
Breakfast Examples:

Poached Eggs:
3	Poached Eggs, discard 2 yolk
1 slice	Bacon
4 oz	Orange Juice or,
½	Grapefruit
1 slice	Wheat Toast
1 t	Jam

Breakfast Ham and Fruit:
5 oz	Breakfast Ham
½	Grapefruit
1	Apple

Cold Cereal:
1 C	All Bran, or (½ C Wheaties, or Special K)
4 oz	Milk, 2%
1 t	Sugar
3 or 4	Strawberries
1	Poached Egg

Hot Cereal:
1 C	Oatmeal
4 oz	Milk, 2%
1 t	Sugar
½ C	Cottage Cheese, 2%

Eating in Restaurants
Lunch Examples:

Chicken:
1	Grilled Chicken Sandwich

Chicken:
3 or 4 oz.	Grilled Chicken Breast
1½ C	Steamed Vegetables, low-glycemic
1	Small Salad
1½ T	Salad Dressing, regular
1	Orange, Tangerine, or 30 Grapes

Salad with Grilled Chicken:
1	Caesar Salad (Have the dressing served separately. Use sparingly.)
3 oz.	Grilled Chicken Breast
1	Orange, Tangerine, or 30 Grapes

Eating in Restaurants
Dinner Examples:

Fish:

3 or 4 oz.	Grilled Fish
1 C	Steamed Vegetables, low-glycemic
1	Salad, side dressing (use sparingly)
1	Orange, Tangerine, or 30 Grapes
1	Glass of Wine
-	Water with a lemon wedge
-	Coffee or Tea

Chicken:

3 or 4 oz.	Grilled Chicken
1 C	Steamed Vegetables, low-glycemic
1	Salad, side dressing (use sparingly)
1	Orange, Tangerine, or 30 Grapes
1	Glass of Wine
-	Water with a lemon wedge
-	Coffee or Tea

Beef:

3 or 4 oz.	Any low-fat steak (Remove all visible fat)
1 C	Steamed Vegetables, low-glycemic rating
1	Salad, side dressing (use sparingly)
1	Orange, Tangerine, or 30 Grapes
1	Glass of Wine
-	Water with a lemon wedge
-	Coffee or Tea

Chinese Foods:

3 to 4 oz.	Teriyaki Chicken
½ to 1 Cup	Rice
1 C	Broccoli (or any low-glycemic vegetable) steamed
1	Glass of Wine
-	Water with a lemon wedge
-	Coffee or Tea

Always drink at least 1 glass of water with each meal. Remember, when dining out you can usually eat 3 to 4 oz. grilled Beef, Fish, or Chicken Breast (what looks like it would fit in the palm of your hand and about as thick as your hand.) (Remove skin or excess fat) Steamed Vegetables (Double the volume of protein if they are low-glycemic vegetables or half the volume of protein if they are high-glycemic vegetables.)

Eating in Restaurants
Dinner Examples:

Deli:

3 to 4 oz.	Sliced Turkey Breast
2 slices	Rye Bread
-	Lettuce and Tomatoes (basically as much as needed)
1 or 2 T	Salad Dressing (Use Sparingly) or
-	Mustard
1	Orange, Tangerine, or 30 Grapes
-	Water with a lemon wedge
-	Coffee or Tea

Italian Foods:

3 to 4 oz.	Grilled Chicken
3 oz.	Pasta
1 C	Steamed Vegetables low-glycemic
1	Small Dinner Salad
1 to 2 T	Salad Dressing, regular
-	Water with a lemon wedge
-	Coffee or Tea
1	Glass of Wine

Japanese Foods:

3 to 4 oz.	Teriyaki Chicken
½ C	Rice
1 C	Steamed Vegetables low-glycemic
1	Small Dinner Salad
1 to 2 T	Salad Dressing (use sparingly)
1	Glass of Wine
-	Water with a lemon wedge
-	Coffee or Tea

Mexican:

3 to 4 oz.	Chicken Fajita's
2	Flour Tortillas
1 to 2 T	Guacamole or Sour Cream
-	Salsa, Tomatoes and Lettuce (basically as much as needed)
1	Glass of Wine
-	Water with a lemon wedge
-	Coffee or Tea

Eating at Fast Food Restaurants
Lunches or Dinners:

These meals are between 2 and 3 block meals

	Protein Blocks	Carb. Blocks	Fat Blocks
Arby's:			
Roast Beef Deluxe	2.5	3.6	3.3
(Take off a little of the bread)			
*Roast Chicken Deluxe	3.4	3.6	2.3
Burger King:			
BK Broiler Chicken Sandwich	2.8	3.6	3.3
Dairy Queen:			
*Grilled Chicken Sandwich	3.5	3.6	2.6
Hardee's:			
*Grilled Chicken Sandwich	3.4	3.7	3.0
Taco Bell:			
Light Taco	1.8	1.2	1.6
Light Taco Supreme	2.0	1.4	1.6
Light Soft Taco	2.1	1.8	1.6
Wendy's:			
*Grilled Chicken Sandwich	3.4	3.8	2.3
Chili, Small	2.7	2.3	2.0

* As you can see, most chicken sandwiches without cheese will be around 3 blocks, as long as they are grilled and not fried in oil. If the sandwich has skin on the chicken, remove the skin before eating the sandwich.

* Spread ¼ teaspoon of butter on the bread if the fat is a block or more less than the carbohydrates or protein. Tear off a little of the bread if it's a bit high in carbohydrates. As long as the PCF's are within the same block number it doesn't matter if the numbers vary.
(Example: 3.1, 3.4, and 3.8, etc.)

Daily Blocked Meals With Snacks

A full day menu for people who eat 12 Blocks per day.

6 weeks of planned meals.

Adjust the meal size or add a snack block to matches your daily block needs.

The recipes for breakfasts, lunches, and snacks are for one person. The amount of groceries given in the shopping lists for breakfasts and lunches is for one person. The amount of groceries given in the shopping list for dinners is for 3 or more people. If you are cooking for less than 3 you can follow the recipe and freeze the extra meals for a later day. If you need more or less than 12 Blocks a day, adjust the meal by choosing an alternative meal or snack from the Alternative Meals starting on page 127 of this book. Or, just pick and chose the meals you want. I just thought it would help you get started on the program a little more comfortably.

Preparation time for most of the dinners takes about 10 or 15 minutes.

If you don't want to eat any of the fruit and/or vegetables I have in the planned meals you can substitute any fruit or vegetables as long as the substitution has about the same PCF's as in the recipe.

Beginning
Weight and Measurements

Name _____
Weight _____
Arm _____
Chest _____
Waist _____
Hips _____
Thigh _____

Name _____
Weight _____
Arm _____
Chest _____
Waist _____
Hips _____
Thigh _____

Name _____
Weight _____
Arm _____
Chest _____
Waist _____
Hips _____
Thigh _____

Name _____
Weight _____
Arm _____
Chest _____
Waist _____
Hips _____
Thigh _____

Staples Shopping List
For Planned Menu

Bay Leaf
Beef Bouillon Cubes
Bread crumbs, plain, toasted
Bread Crumbs, seasoned
Brown Rice (White or Wild)
Brown Sugar
Canola Oil
Cider Vinegar
Cinnamon/Sugar
Cornstarch
Dill Pickles, medium
Fat Free Cooking Spray
Pringles Fat Free Potato Chips
Garlic Powder
Garlic, Granulated
Ground Ginger
Horseradish
Heinz Ketchup
Meat Tenderizer
Miracle Whip, fat free
Miracle Whip, regular
Mustard, Dijon
Mustard, Grey Poupon
Mustard, regular
Olive Oil
Oregano
Paprika
Parmesan Cheese, fat free
Parmesan Cheese, regular
Parsley Flakes
Pepper
Red Wine
Red Wine Vinegar
Pace Salsa
Salt
Slivered Almonds
Soy Sauce
Sugar Free Jell-O, any flavor
Sugar Free Syrup
Sweet Pickles, small
Thyme
Wheat Germ
White Flour
White Rice
White Sugar
White Wine
Worcestershire Sauce

Grocery List
Week 1

Fresh Fruits and Vegetables
1 Green Pepper
2 Lemons
2 qt. Strawberries
Grapefruit
Grapes
3 Tangerines
2 Romaine Lettuce (or mixed greens)
2 Tomato
5 lb. Red Potatoes
Broccoli
Brussels Sprouts
Carrots
Cauliflower
Garlic, Cloves
Onions

Meats
16 oz Ground Beef, 93%
33 oz. Chicken Breasts, (skinless, boneless)
12 oz. Pork Tenderloin
12 oz. Bottom Round Steak
14 3/4 oz. Salmon, canned
Bacon, lean
Turkey Breast, small

Lunch Meats
Canadian Bacon, light
Cooked Ham, 96%
Roast Beef, Deli-Thin 98%
Honey Ham, Deli-thin, 97% lean
Pastrami, Deli-Thin, 98%
Tuna, canned, water pack

Dairy
1 1/2 Doz. Eggs
Butter
2 % Milk
Cheddar Cheese, fat free
American Cheese, fat free, slices
American Cheese, reduced fat, slices
Swiss Cheese slices, fat free
Mozzarella Cheese
Parmesan Cheese, fat free
Whipped Topping, fat free
Orange Juice

Canned Fruits/Vegetables
1-28 oz. Whole Tomatoes
3-15 oz. Tomato Sauce
1 sm. Tomato Sauce
15 oz. Diced Tomatoes, (Italian Style/Herbs)
15 oz. Stewed Tomatoes, (Recipe Style)
2 Mandarin Oranges, light
15 oz. can Asparagus
1 can Green Beans
1 can of Sour Cherries, in water
11 oz can of Corn

Breads/Starches
2 loaves Wheat Bread, Pepperidge Farm, light
Angel Food Cake Mix
Malt-O-Meal
Wheaties
White Rice
2 cans Pringles Fat Free Potato Chips
Angel Hair Spaghetti
English Muffin
English Toasting Bread

Miscellaneous
Jam, any flavor
Miracle Whip, regular
Miracle Whip, fat free
Mustard, Grey Poupon
Dill Pickles, medium
Red Wine Vinegar
Pace Salsa
Beef with Vegetable and Barley Soup
Sugar Free Jell-O
White Wine
Sweet Pickles
Sugar Free Syrup
Fat Free Cooking Spray
Cider Vinegar
Horseradish
Red Wine Vinegar

Oils
Canola Oil
Olive Oil

Planned Meals Week 1

The Alternative Meals Section on Page 127 can be used to substitute any meal I have provided in the 6-week meal plan. Just choose the same number of blocks and make the appropriate changes in the shopping list.

Breakfast - 3 Blocks

Eggs with Ham and Orange Juice

		P	C	F
1	Egg, Whole	6.0	0	5.0
1	Egg White	4.0	0	0
-	Fat Free Cooking Spray	0	0	0
2 slice	Wheat Bread, Pepperidge Farm, light	4.0	14.0	0.5
1½ slices	Cooked Ham, 96% extra lean	7.5	0	1.5
2 T	Pace Salsa	0	3.0	0
4 oz.	Orange Juice	1.0	13.0	0
1 t	Butter	0	0	3.6
		22.5	30.0	10.6
		3.2	3.3	3.5

Spray skillet with a fat free cooking spray and fry the egg and egg white. Remove the eggs to a plate and place the 2 tablespoons of salsa on top of the eggs. Heat ham. Toast the bread and spread one slice with butter and the other with jam.

Lunch - 3 Blocks

Ham & American Cheese Sandwich (Grapes)

		P	C	F
8 slices	Honey Ham, Deli-Thin 97% lean	13.3	2.6	2.0
2 slices	Wheat Bread, Pepperidge Farm, light	4.0	14.0	0.5
1 T	Miracle Whip, regular	0	2.0	7.0
1	Lettuce Leaf, Romaine	0	0	0
1 slice	American Cheese, fat free	5.0	2.0	0
5	Grapes	0	2.5	0
8	Pringles Fat Free Potato Chips	1.0	6.8	0
		23.3	29.9	9.5
		3.3	3.3	3.1

1/2 of any 2 Block Snack

Dinner - 4 Blocks

Steak and Fries for 3		P	C	F
12 oz.	Bottom Round Steak	80.2	0	12.8
1	Garlic Clove, small	0	0	0
½ t	Pepper	0	0	0
-	Salt to taste	0	0	0
1½ T	Canola Oil	0	0	21.0
-	Fat Free Cooking Spray	0	0	0
4	Red Potatoes (about 24 oz.)	7.7	55.7	0
-	Salt	0	0	0
-	Pepper	0	0	0

Mandarin Orange Salad:				
1 C	Romaine Lettuce	3.0	5.0	0
½ C	Mandarin Oranges, light	1.0	16.0	0
15	Grapes	0	7.5	0
2 C	Strawberries, sliced	2.0	14.0	0
1 T	Sugar	0	9.0	0
2 T	Mandarin Orange Salad Dressing	0	6.0	2.2
		93.9	113.2	36.0
		11.8	12.5	12.0
		3.9	4.1	4.0

Mandarin Orange Salad Dressing:
1 t   Canola Oil
3 T   Mandarin Orange liquid, light
1 t   Red Wine Vinegar
1 t   Cider Vinegar
1 t   Sugar

Fries:
   Preheat oven to 500 degrees. Spray 2 large cookie sheets with a fat free cooking spray. Wash potatoes, cut out eyes and slice to ¼" thick. Place potatoes in a bowl and toss with the Canola Oil, salt and pepper. Divide potato slices evenly between pans. Bake about 20 minutes or until tender and lightly browned.

   Cut all visible fat from the steak before weighing. Place steak on a plate and rub with salt, pepper and garlic. Heat Grill on medium high. Grill steak about 14 minutes for medium-rare or until desired doneness, turning once.
   Remove steak to cutting board and thinly slice steak diagonally across the grain.

   Divide and weigh each meal to assure the meals all weigh the same, within a few tenths of an ounce.

   Sugar Free Flavored Gelatin Dessert that has no PCF's can be eaten anytime you feel like snacking.

1/2 of any 2 Block Snack

Breakfast - 3 Blocks

Eggs Benedict   P   C   F

		P	C	F
1	Egg, Whole	6.0	0	5.0
1	Egg, White	4.0	0	0
-	Fat Free Cooking Spray	0	0	0
2 slices	Canadian Bacon, 97% lean	5.0	0.5	0.7
½	English Muffin	2.5	12.5	0.5
3	Potatoes, New, small (6 oz.)	1.9	13.9	0

Hollandaise Sauce:

		P	C	F
1	Egg Yolk	3.0	0	5.0
2 t	Lemon Juice	0	0.8	0
3 T	2% Milk	0	0	0
		22.4	27.7	11.2
		3.2	3.0	3.7

Spray a cool skillet with fat free cooking spray add water and heat. Poach the egg and egg white together. Heat the Canadian Bacon and place on top of English muffin. Add the poached egg to the top of the Canadian bacon then pour the Hollandaise sauce on top.

Sauce:

Place egg yolk and milk in top of double boiler. Cook over boiling water, stirring rapidly, until mixture thickens. (Water in the bottom of the double boiler should not touch the top pan.) Remove pan from water; stir rapidly for 2 minutes. Stir 1 teaspoon of lemon juice at a time. Season with salt and white pepper to taste. Heat again over boiling water, stirring constantly, until thickened. (2 or 3 minutes.) Remove from water at once. If the sauce starts to curdle beat in 1 or 2 teaspoons of boiling water.

Lunch - 3 Blocks

Tuna Melt

		P	C	F
2 oz.	Tuna, water packed	14.9	0	1.0
1 T	Green Onions, chopped	0.1	0.3	0
2 T	Miracle Whip, fat free	0	4.0	0
2 slices	Wheat Bread, Pepperidge Farm, light	4.0	14.0	0.5
1 slices	Swiss Cheese slice, regular	4.0	1.0	5.0
1 t	Butter	0	0	3.6
1	Sweet Pickle, small	0	4.0	0
6	Pringles Fat Free Potato Chips	0.7	6.0	0
2	Strawberry, large	0	1.0	0
		23.7	30.3	10.1
		3.3	3.3	3.3

Spray a cool skillet with fat free cooking spray. Construct the sandwich and grill until golden brown. Serve with fat free potato chips.

1/2 of any 2 Block Snack

Dinner - 4 Blocks

Chicken Cutlet Parmesan in Tomato Sauce for 3		P	C	F
9 oz.	Chicken Breasts, skinless, boneless	58.5	0	3.6
-	Fat Free Cooking Spray	0	0	0
1 ½ T	Olive Oil	0	0	21.0
1 T	Italian Seasoned Bread Crumbs	1.0	4.5	0.4
1 T	Parmesan Cheese, fat free	1.5	4.5	0
1 slice	Mozzarella Cheese (1.5 oz.)	12.0	0	8.0
2 oz	Angel Hair Spaghetti	7.0	40.0	1.0
1 C	Romaine Lettuce	3.0	5.0	0
2 C	Strawberries, sliced	2.0	14.0	1.2
30	Grapes	0	15.0	0
1 T	Mandarin Orange Salad Dressing	0	3.0	1.1
Tomato Sauce:				
1 C	Onion, diced	1.8	11.2	0.2
1	Garlic Clove, minced	0	0	0
15 oz	Diced Tomatoes, Italian Style Herbs	3.0	12.0	0
½ C	Tomato Sauce	1.0	4.0	0
½ t	Sugar	0	2.0	0
2 t	Oregano, dried	0	0	0
		90.8	115.2	36.5
		12.9	12.8	12.1
		4.3	4.2	4.0

Mandarin Orange Salad Dressing: Makes 4 Tablespoons.
- 1 t   Canola Oil
- 3 T   Mandarin Orange liquid, light
- 1 t   Red Wine Vinegar
- 1 t   Cider Vinegar
- 1 t   Sugar

Tomato Sauce:
   Place all tomato sauce ingredients in a saucepan and bring to a boil. Reduce heat to low and simmer about 30 minutes, or until the sauce is thick.
   Spray cool skillet with a fat free cooking spray; add the olive oil and heat. Coat the chicken with the breadcrumbs. (Remove any fat and bone before weighing.)
   Place the breaded chicken into the heated skillet and brown on all sides until the chicken is no longer pink and the juices run clear. Cut the mozzarella cheese into 3 equal portions and place on top of each piece of chicken. Cover and heat until the cheese has melted.
   Cook the spaghetti. Divide and place on a plate. Place a piece of chicken on top, add 1/3 of the sauce. Divide the Parmesan cheese, sprinkle over the sauce and serve.
   Combine salad dressing ingredients, shake well and pour 1 Tablespoon over the lettuce. Mix well, divide and place in bowls. Divide mandarin oranges and place on top of the lettuce.

   Divide and weigh each meal to assure the meals all weigh the same, within a few tenths of an ounce.

   Sugar Free Flavored Gelatin Dessert that has no PCF's can be eaten anytime you feel like snacking.
1/2 of any 2 Block Snack

Breakfast - 2 Blocks

Eggs and Grapefruit

		P	C	F
1	Egg, Whole	6.0	0	5.0
1	Egg, White	4.0	0	0
-	Fat Free Cooking Spray	0	0	0
1 slice	American Cheese, fat free	5.0	2.0	0
1 slice	Wheat Bread, Pepperidge Farm, light	2.0	7.0	0
½ t	Butter	0	0	1.8
½	Grapefruit	1.0	10.0	0
½ t	Sugar	0	2.0	0
		18.0	21.0	6.8
		2.5	2.3	2.2

Spray a cool skillet with fat free cooking spray. Whisk the eggs and add to the heated skillet. Stir eggs occasionally and when almost done tear the American cheese in pieces and stir into the scrambled eggs. Serve with the toast and grapefruit with the sugar.

Lunch - 3 Blocks

Roast Beef Sandwich

		P	C	F
9 slices	Roast Beef, Deli-Thin 98% lean	14.6	2.5	1.0
2 slices	Wheat Bread, Pepperidge Farm, light	4.0	14.0	0.5
2	Lettuce Leaves	0	0	0
1 T	Horseradish	0	0	0
1 T	Miracle Whip, regular	0	2.0	7.0
8	Pringles Fat Free Potato Chips	1.0	6.8	0
1	Dill Pickle, medium	0	1.0	0
		19.6	27.3	8.5
		2.8	2.9	2.8

1/2 of any 2 Block Snack

Dinner - 5 Blocks

Salmon Patties for 3   P   C   F

14¾ oz can	Pink Salmon	84.6	0	30.0
1	Egg, whole	6.0	0	5.0
¼ C	Onions, diced	0.4	2.8	0
1 slice	Wheat Bread, Pepperidge Farm, light cubed	2.0	7.0	0
-	Salt and Pepper to taste	0	0	0
-	Fat Free Cooking Spray	0	0	0
-	White Sauce	4.7	11.5	2.5
1 C	Cauliflower	2.0	5.0	0
1 C	Broccoli	3.0	6.0	0.5
1 T	Butter	0	0	11.0

Dessert:

3 slices	1/12th Angel Food Cake	9.0	90.0	0
1½ C	Strawberries, sliced	1.5	10.5	0
6 T	Cool Whip, fat free	0	9.0	0
		113.2	141.8	49.0
		16.1	15.7	16.3
		5.3	5.2	5.4

White Sauce:

3 T	Water
1 T	Cornstarch
½ C	Milk, 2%
-	Salt, Paprika and Pepper to taste

Bake an Angel Food Cake mix. Divide into 12 equal pieces. The extra pieces can be frozen, or try one of the other recipes that serve Angel Food Cake, strawberries and/or fat free Cool Whip for dessert.

Drain the liquid from the salmon. In a large bowl, place the salmon, egg, diced onions, bread crumbs, and salt and pepper to taste. Shape salmon mixture into 3 equal sized patties. Spray a cool skillet with a Fat Free Cooking Spray and heat. Fry salmon patties until lightly brown.

While the salmon patties are browning, make the white sauce. Stir the cornstarch into the milk, add the rest of the ingredients in a small saucepan, heat and stir over medium heat until thickened. Do not boil.

Steam vegetables and melt the butter over the top. Stir. Divide vegetables by 3 and place on each plate.

When ready to serve, put salmon patties on the plate and pour the white sauce evenly over them. Serve with angel food cake, strawberries and Whipped Topping, fat free.

(You can omit the cool whip and still have a balanced meal.)

Divide and weigh each meal to assure the meals all weigh the same, within a few tenths of an ounce.

Sugar Free Flavored Gelatin Dessert that has no PCF's can be eaten anytime you feel like snacking.

1/2 of any 2 Block Snack

Breakfast - 4 Blocks

Malt-O-Meal

		P	C	F
3 T	Malt-O-Meal (dry)	4.0	26.0	0
1 T	Wheat Germ	2.0	2.0	0.5
1 t	Sugar	0	4.0	0
3 oz	Milk 2%	3.0	4.5	1.2
1	Egg, Whole	6.0	0	5.0
1	Egg, White	4.0	0	0
-	Fat Free Cooking Spray	0	0	0
½ t	Butter	0	0	1.8
1 slice	American Cheese, reduced fat	4.0	3.0	3.0
1 slice	Cooked Ham, 96% extra lean	5.0	0	1.0
		28.0	39.5	12.5
		4.0	4.3	4.1

Cook Malt-O-Meal as directed on package. Sprinkle Wheat Germ and sugar over Malt-O-Meal.

Spray a fat free cooking spray on a cool skillet; add the butter and heat. Scramble the egg and egg whites, pour into heated skillet. When the eggs are almost done tear the cheese into a few pieces and blend into the egg mixture. Stir until cheese is melted. (The ham is larger and thicker than the Deli-Thin slices.) Heat ham in a small skillet and serve.

Lunch - 2 Blocks

B.L.T. with Cheese

		P	C	F
2 slices	Wheat Bread, Pepperidge Farm, light	4.0	14.0	0.5
1½ slices	American Cheese, fat free	7.5	3.0	0
1 leaf	Romaine Lettuce	0	0	0
½	Tomato, medium	0.5	2.0	0
2 slices	Bacon, lean	3.8	0	6.2
2 T	Miracle Whip, fat free	0	4.0	0
		15.8	23.0	6.7
		2.2	2.5	2.2

1/2 of any 2 Block Snack

Dinner - 4 Blocks

Chicken a la Marengo for 3

		P	C	F
12 oz	Chicken Breasts, skinless, boneless	78.0	0	4.8
-	Fat Free Cooking Spray	0	0	0
1½ T	Olive Oil	0	0	21.0
14 oz	Stewed Tomato, recipe style	3.5	24.5	0
1 C	Onions, chopped	1.8	11.2	0.2
¼ t	Garlic Powder	0	0	0
1 t	Parsley	0	0	0
¼ t	Thyme	0	0	0
¼ t	Rosemary	0	0	0
¼ C	White Wine	0	0	0
1	Bay Leaf	0	0	0
-	Salt and Pepper to taste	0	0	0
1½ C	White Rice, cooked	6.0	57.0	0
1 can	Asparagus	7.0	7.0	0
1½ T	Butter	0	0	16.5
10	Grapes	0	5.0	0
¼ C	Mandarin Oranges, light	0.5	8.0	0
1 C	Strawberries, sliced	1.0	7.0	0
		97.8	19.7	42.5
		13.9	13.3	14.1
		4.6	4.4	4.7

Prepare rice as directed on package but omit the butter.

(Remove any fat and bone from the chicken before weighing.)

Lightly spray a cool skillet with a fat free cooking spray. Add the oil. Over medium heat, add the chicken breasts and brown lightly all over. Remove the chicken. Add onion and garlic. Stir until onions are tender.
Return chicken to the skillet. Sprinkle with thyme, parsley and rosemary. Add the stewed tomatoes and juice, wine and bay leaf. Bring to a boil. Reduce heat, cover and simmer for about 20 minutes or until chicken is tender and no longer pink. Serve over rice.

Heat the asparagus. Divide the asparagus and butter by three and place on individual plates. Divide fruit and put into individual bowls.

Divide and weigh each meal to assure the meals all weigh the same, within a few tenths of an ounce.

Sugar Free Flavored Gelatin Dessert that has no PCF's can be eaten anytime you feel like snacking.

1/2 of any 2 Block Snack

Breakfast - 3 Blocks

Wheaties

		P	C	F
1 C	Wheaties	2.7	22.0	0.5
3 oz.	Milk 2%	3.0	4.5	1.8
1 t	Sugar	0	4.0	0
1	Egg, Whole	6.0	0	5.0
½ t	Butter	0	0	1.8
½ slice	American Cheese, fat free	2.5	1.0	0
1½ slices	Cooked Ham, 96% extra lean	7.5	0	1.5
		21.7	31.5	10.6
		3.1	3.5	3.5

Spray a fat free cooking spray on a cool skillet; add the butter and heat. Scramble the egg and pour into the heated skillet. When the egg is almost done tear the cheese into a few pieces and blend into the egg mixture. Stir until cheese is melted. (The ham is larger and thicker than the Deli-Thin slices.) Heat ham in a small skillet and serve. Serve cereal with milk and sugar as a side dish.

Lunch - 3 Blocks

Hot Ham & Swiss

		P	C	F
2 slices	Wheat Bread, Pepperidge Farm, light	4.0	14.0	0.5
2 t	Butter	0	0	7.3
6 slices	Honey Ham, Deli-Thin 97% lean	10.0	2.0	1.5
1 slice	Swiss Cheese, fat free	8.0	1.0	0
1 slice	Onion, sliced thin	0	0	0
1 t	Horseradish	0	0	0
2 t	Mustard	0	0	0
1	Dill Pickle, medium	0	1.0	0
8	Pringles Fat Free Potato chips	1.0	6.8	0
		23.0	24.8	9.8
		3.2	2.7	3.2

Make the sandwich, spread 1-teaspoon of butter on the outside of each slice and grill until golden brown.

Serve with a dill pickle and fat free chips.

1/2 of any 2 Block Snack

Dinner - 4 Blocks

Pork Teriyaki with Orange Salad for 3   P   C   F

		P	C	F
12 oz	Pork Teriyaki Tenderloin	63.0	12.0	12.0
½ C	Carrots, diced	1.0	11.5	0
2 C	Cauliflower	4.0	10.0	0
1½ C	Brussels Sprouts	12.0	40.0	2.6
4 t	Butter	0	0	12.8

Mandarin Orange Salad:

		P	C	F
3 C	Romaine Lettuce	9.0	15.0	0
¼ C	Mandarin Oranges, light	0.5	8.0	0
10	Grapes	0	5.0	0
1 C	Strawberries, sliced	1.0	7.0	0
1 T	Almonds, slivered	3.0	3.0	8.0
2 T	Mandarin Orange Salad Dressing	0	6.0	2.2
		93.5	117.5	37.6
		13.3	13.0	12.5
		4.4	4.3	4.1

Mandarin Orange Salad Dressing: Makes 4 Tablespoons
1 t   Canola Oil
3 T   Mandarin Orange liquid, light
1 t   Red Wine Vinegar
1 t   Cider Vinegar
1 t   Sugar

(Remove any fat and bone before weighing.)

Purchase the Pork Teriyaki Tenderloin and cut it into 12 oz. pieces. (One package usually serves about
3 (3-block meals.) (If you can't find a package of Pork Teriyaki Tenderloin buy Pork Tenderloin and use the Teriyaki Marinade Recipe on page 260 of this book.) Cut the 12 ounces of teriyaki pork into about 1½" thick slices. Grill pork until no longer pink. Steam vegetables, melt the butter over them and divide by 3.

Make the salad dressing, shake well and pour 3 Tablespoons over the lettuce, mix well, divide and place in the bowls. Cut up the grapes and the strawberries. Divide and place on top of lettuce. Divide the mandarin oranges and place on top of lettuce. Put 1 Teaspoon of slivered almonds on each salad.

(You can omit the grapes and strawberries and still have a balanced meal.)

Divide and weigh each meal to assure the meals all weigh the same, within a few tenths of an ounce.

Sugar Free Flavored Gelatin Dessert that has no PCF's can be eaten anytime you feel like snacking.

1/2 of any 2 Block Snack

Breakfast - 3 Blocks

Eggs with Cheese and Bacon

		P	C	F
1	Egg, Whole	6.0	0	5.0
1	Egg White	4.0	0	0
-	Fat Free Cooking Spray	0	0	0
1 Slice	American Cheese, fat free	5.0	2.0	0
½ med.	Tomato, slices	0.5	3.0	0
2 slices	Wheat Toast, Pepperidge Farm, light	4.0	14.0	0.5
1 slice	Bacon, lean	2.7	0	0.3
4 oz.	Orange Juice	1.9	13.0	1.0
2 oz.	Milk 2%	2.0	2.7	1.2
1 t	Butter	0	0	3.6
		24.4	34.7	11.3
		3.4	3.8	3.7

Spray a fat free cooking spray on a cool skillet; add the butter and heat. Scramble the egg and egg white and pour into a heated skillet. When the eggs are almost done tear the cheese into a few pieces and blend into the egg mixture. Stir until cheese is melted. Heat bacon in a small skillet and serve. You can omit the tomato and still have a balanced meal.

Lunch - 3 Blocks

Hot Pastrami

		P	C	F
6 slices	Pastrami, Deli-Thin 98% lean	11.0	1.0	1.0
2 slices	Rye Bread, light	4.0	22.0	2.0
1½ slices	Swiss Cheese, fat free	7.5	4.5	0
2 T	Mustard, Grey Poupon	0	0	0
2 slices	Onion, thin sliced	0	0	0
2 t	Butter	0	0	7.0
1	Dill Pickle, medium	0	1.0	0
		22.5	28.5	10.0
		3.2	3.1	3.3

Spray a cool skillet with fat free cooking spray. Make the sandwich and spread 1-teaspoon of butter on each slice and grill until golden brown. Serve with a dill pickle.

1/2 of any 2 Block Snack

Dinner - 4 Blocks

Texas Hash for 4

16 oz	Ground Beef, 93% lean	84.0	0	24.0
¼ C	Onions, diced	0.4	2.8	0
¼ C	Green Pepper, diced	0.2	2.8	0
28 oz	Whole Tomatoes, canned	7.0	21.0	0
15 oz	Tomato Sauce	7.0	21.0	0
-	Salt and Pepper to taste	0	0	0
1/3 C	White Rice, uncooked	5.3	50.6	0
8 slices	Wheat Bread, Pepperidge Farm, light	16.0	64.0	2.6
2½ T	Butter	0	0	27.5
		119.9	146.2	54.1
		17.1	18.0	18.0
		4.2	4.5	4.5

Brown ground beef with diced onions and green pepper.

Add whole tomatoes and tomato sauce. Season with salt and pepper to taste. Add about 1 Cup of water to the mixture. Stir in the uncooked rice. Cook for 20 minutes, stirring often to keep from sticking.

Makes about 1 3/4 Cups of Texas Hash per person. Serve with 2 slices of bread per blocked meal.

Divide and weigh each meal to assure the meals all weigh the same, within a few tenths of an ounce.

Sugar Free Flavored Gelatin Dessert that has no PCF's can be eaten anytime you feel like snacking.

1/2 of any 2 Block Snack

Breakfast - 3 Blocks

French Toast with Sausage

		P	C	F
1	Egg, Whole	6.0	0	5.0
2	Egg Whites	8.0	0	0
-	Fat Free Cooking Spray	0	0	0
2 slices	Wheat Bread, Pepperidge Farm, light	4.0	14.0	0.5
2 T	Syrup, sugar free	0	6.0	0
1	Breakfast Sausage, 97% fat free	0	0	0
-	(Made with pork and turkey)	7.0	3.0	1.5
1 t	Butter	0	0	3.6
4 oz.	Milk 2%	4.0	5.5	2.5
1 T	Cinnamon Sugar	0	12.0	0
		29.0	40.5	13.1
		4.1	4.5	4.3

Spray a cool skillet with a fat free cooking spray and heat. Stir egg and egg whites, sprinkle a little cinnamon sugar on top of egg mixture and coat the first slice of bread on both sides; place in heated skillet. Sprinkle the remaining cinnamon sugar on top of the eggs and coat the second slice of bread; place in heated skillet. Lightly brown on both sides. Remove bread from skillet and heat the sausage. You can omit the cinnamon sugar and add another tablespoon of syrup.

Any egg that has not been absorbed by the bread should be fried and served on the side.

Lunch - 2 Blocks

Beef with Vegetable & Barley Soup

		P	C	F
½ can	Beef With Vegetable & Barley	6.2	13.7	2.5
1	Hard Boiled Egg	6.0	0	5.0
½ oz	Cheddar Cheese, fat free	4.0	0.5	0
1	Tangerine	0	9.0	0
		16.2	23.2	7.5
		2.3	2.5	2.5

You can substitute any fruit for the tangerine, but make sure it is about the same amount of carbohydrates

1/2 of any 2 Block Snack

Dinner - 4 Blocks

Chicken Breasts with Sour Cherry Sauce for 3   P   C   F

		P	C	F
12 oz	Chicken Breasts (3 breasts, 4 oz. each)	78.0	0	4.8
-	Fat Free Cooking Spray	0	0	0
2 T	Butter	0	0	22.0
½ C	White Wine	0	0	0
5.5 oz.	Sour Cherries in water, (½ can)	3.0	18.0	0
¼ C	Sugar	0	36.0	0
1½ T	Cornstarch	0	10.5	0
½ C	Cherry liquid	0	4.0	0
-	Salt, to taste	0	0	0
11 oz.	Corn (canned)	8.0	40.0	2.0
1 Can	Green Beans	3.5	10.5	0
1 T	Butter	0	0	11.0

Fruit Salad:

¼ C	Mandarin Oranges, light	0.5	8.0	0
1 C	Strawberries	1.0	7.0	0
1 t	Sugar	0	4.0	0
		94.0	134.0	39.8
		13.4	14.8	13.2
		4.4	4.9	4.4

Chicken:
(Remove any fat and bone from the chicken before weighing.)
Spray a cool skillet with a fat free cooking spray. Add 2 T butter and heat. Add the chicken to the hot skillet and brown on both sides. Sprinkle chicken with about ¼ t salt. Add white wine and simmer chicken until chicken is no longer pink and the juice runs clear. (About 10 minutes.)

Meanwhile, in a 2-qt. saucepan, combine cornstarch and sugar.

When chicken is done, using a slotted spoon, transfer to a serving platter. (Cover to keep warm.)

Strain the chicken liquid from skillet and add to the cornstarch mixture. Heat to a boil, stirring constantly, until sauce thickens. Stir in the pitted cherries. Cook until cherries are heated through.

Divide the cherries and sauce equally and spoon over the chicken on the platter. Serve with heated vegetables and fruit salad.

Divide and weigh each meal to assure the meals all weigh the same, within a few tenths of an ounce.

You can omit the fruit salad and still have a balanced meal.

Sugar Free Flavored Gelatin Dessert that has no PCF's can be eaten anytime you feel like snacking.

1/2 of any 2 Block Snack

Weight and Measurements
Results Week 1

Name _____
Weight _____
Arm _____
Chest _____
Waist _____
Hips _____
Thigh _____

Name _____
Weight _____
Arm _____
Chest _____
Waist _____
Hips _____
Thigh _____

Name _____
Weight _____
Arm _____
Chest _____
Waist _____
Hips _____
Thigh _____

Name _____
Weight _____
Arm _____
Chest _____
Waist _____
Hips _____
Thigh _____

Grocery List
Week 2

Fresh Fruits and Vegetables
Grapes
1 Lemon
5 C Strawberries
2 Green Peppers
2 Romaine Lettuce (or mixed greens)
2 Tomato
Broccoli
Brussels Sprouts
Carrots
Cauliflower
Garlic Cloves
Green Onions
Onions
Red Potatoes
Tarragon, fresh

Meats
16 oz Ground Beef, 93%
9 oz Top Sirloin, lean
24 oz. Chicken Breasts, skinless, boneless
12 oz. Pork Tenderloin
24 oz Orange Roughy (or any white fish)
Tuna, Albacore, water-packed, canned

Lunch Meats
Breakfast Sausage 97% (fat free made with pork and turkey)
Canadian Bacon, lean
Cooked Ham, 96%
Honey Ham, Deli-Thin, 97% lean
Chicken Breast, Deli Thin 97% lean
Bacon

Dairy
1 Doz. Eggs
Butter
2 % Milk
Cottage Cheese 2%
American Cheese, fat free, slices
American Cheese, reduced fat, slices
Swiss Cheese slices, fat free
Mozzarella Cheese reg.
Parmesan Cheese, fat free
Cool Whip, fat free
Orange Juice

Canned Fruits/Vegetables
1-28 oz. Whole Tomatoes
3-15 oz. Tomato Sauce
15 oz Italian Tomatoes
3 Mandarin Oranges, light
15 oz. cans Asparagus
1 can Green Beans
2-11 oz can Corn
Vegetarian Vegetable Soup

Breads/Starches
2 loaves Wheat Bread, Pepperidge Farm, light
Oatmeal
Lasagna Noodles
Angel Food Cake Mix
Smart Start Cereal
English Toasting Bread
Pringles Fat Free Potato Chips
White Rice

Nuts/Seeds
Almonds slivered

Miscellaneous
Jam, any flavor
Sweet Pickles, small
Dill Pickles
Fat free Cooking Spray
Worcestershire Sauce
Dark Raisins
Heinz Ketchup
Brown Sugar
Red Wine
Pace Salsa
Cider Vinegar
White Wine
White Wine Vinegar
Cinnamon/Sugar
Sugar Free Jell-O
Soy Sauce
Sugar Free Syrup
Miracle Whip fat free
Miracle Whip regular

Oils:
Olive Oil
Canola Oil

Spices:
Basil
Oregano
Thyme
Parsley Flakes
Bay Leaf
Garlic, Granulated
Garlic Powder
Onion Salt

Planned Meals Week 2

Breakfast - 3 Blocks

Eggs with Ham and Orange Juice

		P	C	F
1	Egg, Whole	6.0	0	5.0
-	Fat Free Cooking Spray	0	0	0
2 slice	Wheat Bread, Pepperidge Farm, light	4.0	14.0	0.5
1½ slices	Cooked Ham, 96% extra lean	7.5	0	1.5
2 T	Pace Salsa	0	3.0	0
4 oz.	Orange Juice	1.0	13.0	0
1 t	Butter	0	0	3.6
		22.5	30.0	10.6
		3.2	3.3	3.5

Spray a fat free cooking spray on a cool skillet and heat. Scramble the egg and pour into heated skillet. (The ham is larger and thicker than the Deli-Thin slices.) Heat ham in a small skillet and serve. Heat the salsa and pour over egg. Toast the bread and spread the butter on the toast.

Lunch - 3 Blocks

Tuna Sandwich

		P	C	F
2.5 oz.	Tuna, Albacore, water packed	18.7	0	1.3
2 slices	Wheat Bread, Pepperidge Farm, light	4.0	14.0	0.5
2 T	Onion, diced	0	1.4	0.2
2	Lettuce Leaves	0	0	0
1 T	Miracle Whip, regular	0	2.0	7.0
1	Sweet Pickle, small	0	4.0	0
8	Pringles Fat Free Potato Chips	1.0	6.8	0
		23.7	28.2	9.3
		3.3	3.1	3.1

Mix the tuna with the diced onions and Miracle Whip and spread on one slice of bread. Place the lettuce on top and put the other slice of bread on top. Serve with a sweet pickle and chips.

(A 9-ounce can of tuna makes 3 sandwiches)
(After draining, there is 7.5 oz of tuna.)

1/2 of any 2 Block Snack

Dinner - 4 Blocks

Grilled Orange Roughy and Apple Cole Slaw for 3

		P	C	F
12 oz.	Orange Roughy (or any other white fish)	63.7	0	3.9
-	Fat Free Cooking Spray	0	0	0
1½ T	Butter	0	0	16.5
1½ t	Lemon Juice	0	0.5	0
3 T	Miracle Whip, fat free	0	6.0	0
1 T	Sweet Pickle Relish	0.1	5.3	0.1
2 C	Cabbage, shredded	2.0	8.0	0
½	Apple, medium chopped	0	8.7	0
2 T	Raisins, dark	0.7	15.2	0
1	Celery Stalk, chopped	0	2.0	0
3 T	Miracle Whip, fat free	0	6.0	0
½ T	Milk 2%	0	0	0
½ T	Cider Vinegar	0	0.4	0
1 Can	Asparagus	7.0	7.0	0
11 oz.	Corn (canned)	8.0	40.0	2.0
1 T	Butter	0	0	11.0
		81.5	99.1	33.5
		11.6	11.0	11.51
		3.8	3.6	3.7

    Grate cabbage and put in a large bowl. Chop apples and celery and place on top of grated cabbage. Mix the dressing, pour over the slaw, mix well, and set aside.

    Mix miracle whip and sweet pickle relish and set aside. (You can omit the 3 Tablespoons of Miracle Whip and the sweet pickle relish and add 3 Tablespoons of Ketchup and still be in balance.)

    Thaw frozen fish in milk, or if it's fresh, soak in the milk until ready to cook. Discard the left over milk. Spray a cool skillet with a fat free cooking spray and add 1½ teaspoon of butter. Heat skillet; sprinkle the fish with salt and pepper. Fry fish until the fish flakes. (7 to 10 minutes.)

    Steam vegetables, divide the remaining butter and melt over top. Serve with Apple Cole slaw. Divide the raisins and sprinkle on top of each bowl of coleslaw when ready to serve.

    Divide and weigh each meal to assure the meals all weigh the same, within a few tenths of an ounce.

    Sugar Free Flavored Gelatin Dessert that has no PCF's can be eaten anytime you feel like snacking.

1/2 of any 2 Block Snack

Breakfast - 3 Blocks

Sausage and Eggs with Cantaloupe

		P	C	F
1	Egg, Whole	4.0	0	5.0
1	Egg White	4.0	0	0
-	Fat Free Cooking Spray	0	0	0
2 T	Pace Salsa	0	3.0	0
2	Breakfast Sausage, 97% fat free	0	0	0
-	(Made with pork and turkey)	7.0	3.0	1.5
1 slice	Wheat Bread, Pepperidge Farm, light	1.0	7.0	0
½ t	Butter	0	0	1.8
1 Cup	Cantaloupe	1.4	13.4	0.4
		17.4	26.4	8.7
		2.4	2.9	2.9

Spray a fat free cooking spray on a cool skillet; add the butter and heat. Whisk the egg and egg white and pour into heated skillet. Heat the salsa and pour over the scrambled eggs. Heat the sausage according to package directions. Toast the bread and spread with the butter. Cube cantaloupe and serve in a salad bowl.

Lunch - 3 Blocks

Vegetarian Vegetable Soup & Ham Sandwich

		P	C	F
½ Can	Vegetarian Vegetable	3.7	20.0	1.2
2 slices	Wheat Bread, Pepperidge Farm, light	2.0	7.0	0
1½ slices	American Cheese, fat free	7.5	3.0	0
2 slices	Cooked Ham, 96% extra lean	10.0	0	3.0
1 T	Miracle Whip, regular	0	2.0	7.0
-	Salt and Pepper to taste	0	0	0
		23.2	32.0	11.2
		3.3	3.5	3.7

If you would prefer your ham sandwich hot, spray a cool skillet with fat free cooking spray, put the sandwich together and grill until bread is browned on both sides and the cheese has melted.

1/2 of any 2 Block Snack

Dinner - 4 Blocks

Steak and Potatoes for 3   P   C   F
9 oz.   Top Sirloin, lean (3 oz. each)   77.4   0   17.3
3 T   Worcestershire Sauce   0   0   0
½ t   Onion Salt   0   0   0
½ t   Garlic Powder   0   0   0
1 t   Meat Tenderizer   0   0   0

7   Potatoes, Red small chunks (14 oz.)   4.6   32.6   0
1 C   Broccoli   3.0   6.0   0.5
1 C   Carrots, cut in chunks   2.0   23.0   0
2 T   Butter   0   0   22.0

Mandarin Orange Salad:
2 C   Romaine Lettuce   6.0   10.0   0
¼ C   Mandarin Oranges, light   0.5   8.0   0
20   Grapes   0   10.0   0
1½ C   Strawberries, sliced   1.5   14.0   0
2 t   Sugar   0   8.0   0
2 T   Mandarin Orange Salad Dressing   0   6.0   2.2
                                                                            95.0   117.6   42.0
                                                                            13.5   13.0   14.0
                                                                            4.5   4.3   4.6

Mandarin Orange Salad Dressing:
1 t   Canola Oil
3 T   Mandarin Orange liquid, light
1 t   Red Wine Vinegar
1 t   Cider Vinegar
1 t   Sugar

    Cut all visible fat from the steak before weighing. Cut into 3 equal pieces, 3 oz. each. Sprinkle meat tenderizer, garlic powder, and onion salt. Rub into meat. Using a fork, stab the spices deep into the meat. Pour Worcestershire sauce on each piece and stab again. Grill the meat.
    Steam the potatoes, broccoli and carrots in separate sides of the steamer. (Making it easier to divide when ready to serve.) Melt the butter over the steamed vegetables and serve.
    Combine salad dressing ingredients, shake well and pour 2 Tablespoons over the lettuce. Mix well, divide and place in bowls. Cut Grapes in half. Dice the strawberries, put 2t sugar on them and mix well. Divide mandarin oranges, strawberries and grapes. Place on top of the lettuce. **(You can omit the grapes or mandarin oranges and still have a balanced meal.)**

    Divide and weigh each meal to assure the meals all weigh the same, within a few tenths of an ounce.
    Sugar Free Flavored Gelatin Dessert that has no PCF's can be eaten anytime you feel like snacking.

1/2 of any 2 Block Snack

Breakfast - 4 Blocks

Omelet with Ham and Orange Juice

		P	C	F
1	Egg, Whole	6.0	0	5.0
2	Egg Whites	8.0	0	0
-	Fat Free Cooking Spray	0	0	0
1 slice	Cooked Ham, 96% extra lean, diced	5.0	0	1.0
1 T	Green Pepper, diced	0	0.7	0
1 T	Onion, diced	0.1	0.7	0
2 T	Cheddar Cheese, shredded, fat free	4.5	0.5	0
1 T	Celery, diced	0	0	0
2 slices	Wheat Toast, Pepperidge Farm, light	4.0	14.0	0.5
3 oz.	Milk 2%	3.0	4.5	1.2
4 oz.	Orange Juice	0.8	13.0	0
1½ t	Butter	0	0	5.4
1 t	Jam, light	0	3.0	0
		31.4	36.4	13.1
		4.4	4.0	4.3

Dice all vegetables and set aside. Spray a cool skillet with fat free cooking spray and heat. Whisk the eggs and pour into the skillet. Add the vegetables, ham and cheese on one side of the eggs. Fold the other side of the eggs over the vegetables. Toast the bread, spread butter on one slice and jam on the other.

Lunch - 2 Blocks

Grilled Ham and Cheese Sandwich

		P	C	F
2 slices	Wheat Bread, Pepperidge Farm, light	4.0	14.0	0.5
2 slices	American Cheese, reduced fat	8.0	4.0	6.0
½ T	Miracle Whip, fat free	0	1.0	0
1 slice	Cooked Ham, 96% extra lean	5.0	0	1.0
4	Pringles Fat Free Potato Chips	0.5	3.4	0
-	Salt and Pepper to taste	0	0	0
		17.5	22.4	7.5
		2.5	2.5	2.5

Spray a cool skillet with fat free cooking spray. Construct the sandwich, add salt and pepper and grill until golden brown. Serve with 4 fat free potato chips.

1/2 of any 2 Block Snack

Dinner - 4 Blocks

Garlic Chicken with Angel Food Cake for 3		P	C	F
12 oz.	Chicken Breasts, skinless, boneless	78.0	0	4.8
3	Garlic Cloves, peeled	0.3	1.4	0
-	Fat Free Cooking Spray	0	0	0
½ T	Olive Oil	0	0	7.7
1 T	White Wine Vinegar	0	0.6	0
¼ C	Chicken Broth	0.2	0.2	0.3
1½ T	Butter	0	0	16.5
½ T	Fresh Tarragon, chopped	0	0	0
1 C	Cauliflower, raw	2.0	5.0	0
½ C	Snow Peas, raw	2.0	6.0	0
1 T	Butter	0	0	11.0
Dessert:				
3 slices	1/12th Angel Food Cake	9.0	90.0	0
1½ C	Strawberries, sliced	1.5	10.5	0
6 T	Cool Whip, fat free	0	9.0	0
		93.0	122.7	40.3
		13.2	13.6	13.4
		4.4	4.5	4.4

 Bake an Angel Food Cake mix. Divide into 12 equal pieces. (The extra pieces can be frozen, or make one of the other recipes that serve Angel Food Cake for dinner tomorrow night) Serve with strawberries and/or fat free Whipped Topping for dessert.
 (Remove any fat and bone before weighing.)
 Spray a cool skillet with a fat free cooking spray, and add the olive oil and butter. Brown chicken on all sides. Add the garlic cloves, white wine vinegar, chicken broth and tarragon. Cook over low heat until the chicken is no longer pink and the juices run clear.

 Steam Vegetables, remove from steamer, melt 1 Tablespoon of butter over them, and blend well. Divide into 3 portions. (You don't have to worry if the individual vegetables are divided equally as they have about the same PCF's.)

 Angel food cake with strawberries and Cool Whip, fat free, for dessert.

 (You can substitute 1 Cup of canned sliced Peaches, light, 2 fresh peaches, or ½ C mandarin oranges, for the strawberries, and still be balanced. Or try another substitution.)

 Divide and weigh each meal to assure the meals all weigh the same, within a few tenths of an ounce

 Sugar Free Flavored Gelatin Dessert that has no PCF's can be eaten anytime you feel like snacking.

1/2 of any 2 Block Snack

Breakfast - 3 Blocks

Smart Start Cereal		P	C	F
2/3 C	Smart Start Cereal	2.0	27.3	0.3
3 oz.	Milk 2%	3.0	4.5	1.8
-	Fat Free Cooking Spray	0	0	0
1	Egg, Whole	6.0	0	5.0
2	Egg, Whites	8.0	0	0
1 t	Butter	0	0	3.6
½ slice	American Cheese, fat free	2.7	1.0	0
1 slice	Canadian Bacon, lean	2.7	0	0.3
		24.4	32.8	11.0
		3.4	3.6	3.6

Spray a fat free cooking spray on a cool skillet; add the butter and heat. Scramble the egg and egg whites, and pour into heated skillet. When the eggs are almost done tear the cheese into a few pieces and blend into the egg mixture. Stir until cheese is melted. Heat the Canadian bacon in a small skillet. Serve with the Cereal and milk.

Lunch - 3 Blocks

Hot Ham & Swiss		P	C	F
2 slices	Wheat Bread, Pepperidge Farm, light	4.0	14.0	0.5
2 t	Butter	0	0	7.3
6 slices	Honey Ham, Deli-Thin 97% lean	10.0	2.0	1.5
1 slice	Swiss Cheese, fat free	8.0	1.0	0
1 slice	Onion, sliced thin	0	0	0
1 t	Horseradish	0	0	0
2 t	Mustard	0	0	0
1	Dill Pickle, medium	0	1.0	0
8	Pringles Fat Free Potato Chips	1.0	6.8	0
		23.0	24.8	9.8
		3.2	2.7	3.2

Spray a cool skillet with fat free cooking spray. Make the sandwich. Spread 1 teaspoon of butter on each slice of bread and grill until golden brown. Serve sandwich with the dill pickle and chips on the side.

1/2 of any 2 Block Snack

Dinner - 4 Blocks

Cheesy Orange Roughy for 3

		P	C	F
12 oz.	Orange Roughy (or any other white fish)	64.0	0	4.0
3 T	Parmesan Cheese, fat free	4.5	13.5	0
-	Fat Free Cooking Spray	0	0	0
1 T	Butter	0	0	11.0
6 T	Heinz Ketchup	0	24.0	0
1 C	Brussels Sprouts	6.0	20.0	1.0
1 C	Cauliflower	2.0	5.0	0
1 T	Butter	0	0	11.0

Mandarin Orange Salad:

		P	C	F
3 C	Romaine Lettuce	9.0	15.0	0
¼ C	Mandarin Oranges, light	0.5	8.0	0
15	Grapes	0	7.5	0
1 C	Strawberries, sliced	1.0	7.0	0
1 T	Almond slivered	3.0	3.0	8.0
2 T	Mandarin Orange Salad Dressing	0	6.0	2.2
		90.0	109.0	37.2
		12.8	12.1	12.4
		4.2	4.0	4.1

Thaw fish in milk. Discard the left over milk. Spray a cool skillet with a fat free cooking spray and add 1 Tablespoon of butter. Heat skillet, sprinkle the fish with salt and pepper and fry fish until it flakes, (7 to 10 min.)

Sprinkle Parmesan cheese over fish, cover and keep warm.

Steam Brussels sprouts and cauliflower. Melt butter over top, divide and serve.

Combine salad dressing ingredients, shake well and pour 2 Tablespoons of dressing over the lettuce, mix well, divide and place in bowls. Cut grapes in half. Dice strawberries. Divide mandarin oranges, strawberries and grapes and place on top of lettuce.

(You can omit strawberries or grapes and still have a balanced meal.)
(You can omit ketchup and add 9 Tablespoons of Miracle Whip, fat free, or a combination, and still be balanced.)

Divide and weigh each meal to assure the meals all weigh the same, within a few tenths of an ounce.

Sugar Free Flavored Gelatin Dessert that has no PCF's and can be eaten anytime you feel like snacking.

1/2 of any 2 Block Snack

Breakfast - 3 Blocks

Eggs with Ham and Cheese

		P	C	F
1	Egg, Whole	6.0	0	5.0
-	Fat Free Cooking Spray	0	0	0
1 Slice	American Cheese, fat free	5.0	2.0	0
1 slice	English Toasting Bread	3.0	14.0	1.0
1 slice	Cooked Ham, 96% extra lean	5.0	0	1.0
2 oz	Milk 2%	2.0	2.7	1.2
3 oz.	Orange Juice	0.7	9.7	0
½ t	Butter	0	0	1.8
		21.7	28.4	10.0
		3.1	3.1	3.3

Spray a cool skillet with fat free cooking spray and heat. Whisk the egg and pour into the skillet. When egg is almost done tear up the cheese and stir into the egg. Heat the ham and serve.

Lunch - 2 Blocks

Egg Salad Sandwich

		P	C	F
2 slices	Wheat Bread, Pepperidge Farm, light	4.0	14.0	0.5
1	Egg, Whole	6.0	0	5.0
1	Egg, White	4.0	0	0
2 T	Miracle Whip, fat free	0	4.0	0
½ t	Butter	0	0	1.8
5	Grapes	0	2.5	0
		14.0	20.5	7.3
		2.0	2.2	2.4

Put cold water in a small saucepan. Add the egg s, cover and cook over medium high heat until the water boils. Remove the pan from the heat and let set for 20 minutes. Shell the eggs but throw away one egg yolk. Chop egg and egg white. Stir in the miracle whip. Spread bread with the butter and put on the egg salad.

1/2 of any 2 Block Snack

Dinner - 5 Blocks

Pork Roast and Vegetables for 3   P   C   F

		P	C	F
12 oz.	Pork Tenderloin	68.0	0	20.0
-	Fat Free Cooking Spray	0	0	0
1½ T	Butter	0	0	16.5
1 C	Onions, diced	1.8	11.2	0.2
6	Potatoes, New Red small (12 oz.)	3.9	27.9	0
1½ C	Carrots, diced (5.5 oz.)	2.0	23.0	0

Mandarin Orange Salad:

		P	C	F
1 C	Romaine Lettuce	3.0	5.0	0
¼ C	Mandarin Oranges, light	0.5	8.0	0
10	Grapes	0	5.0	0
1 C	Strawberries, sliced	1.0	7.0	0
1 T	Mandarin Orange Salad Dressing	0	3.0	1.1
12 oz.	Milk, 2% (4 oz. each)	12.0	16.5	7.5
3 slices	Wheat Bread, Pepperidge Farm, light	7.0	22.0	1.0
		99.2	128.6	46.3
		14.1	14.2	15.4
		4.7	4.7	5.1

Mandarin Orange Salad Dressing: Makes 4 T of dressing.
1 t   Canola Oil
3 T   Mandarin Orange liquid, light
1 t   Red Wine Vinegar
1 t   Cider Vinegar
1 t   Sugar

    Spray an electric skillet with a fat free cooking spray and add 1½ Tablespoons of butter. (Remove as much fat and bone as possible before weighing pork roast.)
    Sprinkle meat lightly with salt and pepper. Brown the pork roast on all sides.
    Cut the onion into about 8 pieces. Peel potatoes and carrots and cut into bite size pieces. Add the onions, potatoes, and carrots to the skillet. Cook over low heat, stirring often, until the vegetables are tender and the pork roast is no longer pink; keep adding water to keep the food from burning.

    Eat one slice of bread per serving. **Don't put any butter on the bread.**

    Combine salad dressing ingredients, shake well and pour 1 Tablespoon of dressing over the lettuce, mix well, divide and place in bowls. Divide mandarin oranges, strawberries, and grapes, place on top of lettuce.
    (You can omit the grapes and/or strawberries and still have a balanced meal.)
    Divide and weigh each meal to assure the meals all weigh the same, within a few tenths of an ounce.
    Sugar Free Flavored Gelatin Dessert that has no PCF's and can be eaten anytime you feel like snacking.
1/2 of any 2 Block Snack

Breakfast - 3 Blocks

Oatmeal

		P	C	F
½ C	Oatmeal, dry	6.0	25.0	2.0
3 oz.	Milk 2%	3.0	4.5	1.8
1 t	Sugar	0	4.0	0
1	Egg, Whole	6.0	0	5.0
1	Egg, White	4.0	0	0
½ t	Butter	0	0	1.8
1 slice	American Cheese, fat free	5.0	2.0	0
		24.0	35.5	10.6
		3.4	3.9	3.5

Cook the oatmeal according to the directions on the package.

Meanwhile, spray a cool skillet with fat free cooking spray; add the butter and heat. Whisk the egg and egg white and pour into the skillet. When the eggs are almost done tear up the cheese and blend into the eggs.

Serve cheesy eggs on the side with the oatmeal.

Lunch - 3 Blocks

Tuna Melt

		P	C	F
2 oz.	Tuna, water packed	14.9	0	1.0
1 T	Green Onions, chopped	0.1	0.3	0
2 T	Miracle Whip, fat free	0	4.0	0
2 slices	Wheat Bread, Pepperidge Farm, light	4.0	14.0	0.5
1 slices	Swiss Cheese slice, regular	4.0	1.0	5.0
1 t	Butter	0	0	3.6
1	Sweet Pickle, small	0	4.0	0
6	Pringles Fat Free Potato Chips	0.7	6.0	0
2	Strawberry, large	0	1.0	0
		23.7	30.3	10.1
		3.3	3.3	3.3

Spray a cool skillet with fat free cooking spray.

Weigh out 2 ounces of tuna; add the green onions and miracle whip. Blend well. Spread the tuna salad on the bread; add the cheese and then spread the butter on the outside of the slices and fry in the skillet until golden brown. Serve with a sweet pickle, strawberries, and fat free chips.

1/2 of any 2 Block Snack

Dinner - 5 Blocks

Lasagna for 6   P   C   F

Amount	Ingredient	P	C	F
16 oz.	Ground Beef 93% lean	84.0	0	24.0
½ C	Onions, diced	0.9	5.6	0.1
2	Garlic Cloves	0	0	0
1 T	Brown Sugar	0	12.0	0
2 T	Oregano	0	0	0
1/8 t	Thyme	0	0	0
¼ C	Parsley Flakes	0	0	0
1	Bay Leaf	0	0	0
28 oz.	Whole Tomatoes (canned)	7.0	21.0	0
45 oz.	Tomato Sauce	21.0	42.0	0
8 oz.	Mozzarella Cheese, reduced fat	72.0	8.0	16.0
4.5 oz.	Lasagna Noodles (6)	15.7	90.0	2.2
12 slices	Wheat Bread, Pepperidge Farm, light	28.0	88.0	4.0
4½ T	Butter	0	0	49.5
½ t	Garlic, Granulated	0	0	0
		228.6	266.6	95.8
		32.6	29.6	31.9
		5.4	4.9	5.3

Heat oven to 350 degrees.

Brown meat, onions and garlic in skillet. Add the next 7 ingredients and simmer about 2 hours or until sauce is thick. (Use spices to suit your own taste.) Discard Bay Leaf.

Cook lasagna noodles. Slice the cheese in 24 fairly equal pieces, weigh and divide into 6 equal portions. (About 1.4 oz. on each layer of the 6 portions.) Cover the bottom of a rectangle casserole dish with a thin layer of sauce. Place 3 lasagna noodles on sauce. Divide the rest of the sauce in about half. Put one half the sauce and half the cheese on top of the sauce. Add the rest of the noodles, top with the remaining sauce and cheese. (12 slices of cheese per layer. 4 slices of cheese per serving.)
Bake for about 20 minutes or until the cheese is melted.
While the lasagna is baking, toast 12 slices of bread. (2 for each person.) Stir garlic powder into the butter and spread on the toast.
Remove the lasagna pan from the oven and let stand for about 10 minutes before serving.
Divide the lasagna into six portions. If all the lasagna is not served at the meal freeze in individual containers for future meal or serve for dinner tomorrow night.

Divide and weigh each meal to assure the meals all weigh the same, within a few tenths of an ounce.
Sugar Free Flavored Gelatin Dessert that has no PCF's and can be eaten anytime you feel like snacking.

1/2 of any 2 Block Snack

Breakfast - 3 Blocks

French Toast with Ham

		P	C	F
1	Egg, Whole	6.0	0	5.0
1	Egg White	4.0	0	0
-	Fat Free Cooking Spray	0	0	0
2 slices	Wheat Bread, Pepperidge Farm, light	4.0	14.0	0.5
2 T	Syrup, sugar free	0	6.0	0
1 slice	Cooked Ham, 96% extra lean	5.0	0	1.0
½ t	Butter	0	0	1.8
4 oz.	Milk 2%	4.0	5.5	2.5
1½ t	Cinnamon Sugar	0	6.0	0
		23.0	31.5	10.8
		3.2	3.5	3.6

    Spray a cool skillet with a fat free cooking spray and heat. Whisk egg and egg white, sprinkle a little cinnamon sugar on top of egg mixture and coat the first slice of bread on both sides; place in heated skillet. Sprinkle the remaining cinnamon sugar on top of the eggs and coat the second slice of bread; place in heated skillet. Lightly brown on both sides. Heat the Canadian bacon in a small skillet.

    Remove bread from skillet, spread on the butter and pour 1-tablespoon of syrup on each slice. Serve with the Canadian bacon. You can omit the cinnamon sugar and add another tablespoon of syrup. Any egg not absorbed by the bread should be fried and served as a side dish.

Lunch - 3 Blocks

Hot Ham & Swiss

		P	C	F
2 slices	Wheat Bread, Pepperidge Farm, light	4.0	14.0	0.5
2 t	Butter	0	0	7.3
6 slices	Honey Ham, Deli-Thin 97% lean	10.0	2.0	1.5
1 slice	Swiss Cheese, fat free	8.0	1.0	0
1 slice	Onion, sliced thin	0	0	0
1 t	Horseradish	0	0	0
2 t	Mustard	0	0	0
1	Dill Pickle, medium	0	1.0	0
8	Pringles Fat Free Potato Chips	1.0	6.8	0
		23.0	24.8	9.8
		3.2	2.7	3.2

    Spray a cool skillet with fat free cooking spray and set aside. Make the sandwich; spread 1-teaspoon of butter on the top of each slice of bread and fry until golden brown. Serve with a dill pickle and chips.

1/2 of any 2 Block Snack

Dinner - 4 Blocks

Chicken Cacciatore for 3

Amount	Ingredient	P	C	F
12 oz.	Chicken Breasts, skinless, boneless	77.8	0	4.8
-	Fat Free Cooking Spray	0	0	0
-	Salt and Pepper to taste	0	0	0
2 T	Olive Oil	0	0	28.0
½ C	Onions, diced	09	5.6	0
1 C	Green Pepper, diced	08	11.2	0.2
½ t	Garlic Powder	0	0	0
½ C	Red Wine	0	0	0
½ t	Oregano	0	0	0
½ t	Basil	0	0	0
1 t	Parsley	0	0	0
14.5 oz.	Italian Tomatoes, canned	3.5	17.5	0
1 Can	Green Beans	1.0	10.5	0
1 t	Butter	0	0	3.6
1½ C	White Rice, cooked	6.0	57.0	0

Mandarin Orange Salad:

Amount	Ingredient	P	C	F
2 C	Romaine Lettuce	6.0	10.0	0
6	Grapes	0	2.5	0
1 C	Strawberries, sliced	1.0	7.0	0
1 T	Mandarin Orange Salad Dressing	0	3.0	1.1
		97.0	124.3	37.7
		13.8	13.8	12.5
		4.6	4.6	4.1

Mandarin Orange Salad Dressing: Makes 4 Tablespoons

1 t	Canola Oil
3 T	Mandarin Orange liquid, light
1 t	Red Wine Vinegar
1 t	Cider Vinegar
1 t	Sugar

Prepare rice as directed on package but omit the butter.

Lightly spray a cool skillet with a fat free cooking spray; add the oil and heat. Sprinkle chicken with salt and pepper. Fry about 4 minutes or until chicken is lightly browned on both sides. Add the onions, green pepper, and garlic powder to the skillet. Stir in wine, tomatoes, oregano, basil and parsley. Bring to a boil, reduce heat to medium low, cover and simmer for about 30 minutes or until chicken is tender and no longer pink. Serve over rice. Heat green beans and divide into 3 portions.

Combine salad dressing ingredients, shake well and pour 1 Tablespoon over the lettuce, mix well, divide and place in bowls. Divide grapes and strawberries, place on top of lettuce. (You can omit the strawberries and/or grapes and still be balanced.)

Divide and weigh each meal to assure the meals all weigh the same, within a few tenths of an ounce.
Sugar Free Flavored Gelatin Dessert that has no PCF's can be eaten anytime you feel like snacking.

1/2 of any 2 Block Snack

Weight and Measurements
Results Week 2

Name _____
Weight _____
Arm _____
Chest _____
Waist _____
Hips _____
Thigh _____

Name _____
Weight _____
Arm _____
Chest _____
Waist _____
Hips _____
Thigh _____

Name _____
Weight _____
Arm _____
Chest _____
Waist _____
Hips _____
Thigh _____

Name _____
Weight _____
Arm _____
Chest _____
Waist _____
Hips _____
Thigh _____

Grocery List
Week 3

Fresh Fruits and Vegetables
7 Peaches
1 Lemon
1 qt. Strawberries
Grapes
2 Green Peppers
2 Romaine Lettuce (or mixed greens)
1 Tomato
5 lb. Red Potatoes
Broccoli
Cabbage
Cauliflower
Garlic, Cloves
Onions
Green Onions
Pearl Onions

Meats
10.5 oz Fillet of Sole
12 oz Large Shrimp
10 oz Top Sirloin Steak
24 oz Chicken Breasts boneless, skinless
16 oz Bottom Round
2 Tuna, Albacore, water packed
Turkey Breast, small

Lunch Meats
Canadian Bacon, lean
Cooked Ham, 96%
Honey Ham, Deli-thin, 97% lean
Bacon

Dairy
1 Doz. Eggs
Butter
2 % Milk
Cottage Cheese 2%
American Cheese, (reduced fat, slices)
Parmesan Cheese (fat free)
Swiss Cheese, fat free
Swiss Cheese regular
Feta Cheese
Gruyere Cheese
Monterey Jack Cheese
Cool Whip, fat free
Orange Juice
Sour Cream, fat free

Canned Fruits/Vegetables
16 oz Whole Tomatoes
4.5 oz can Mushrooms
Tomato Paste
1 can Beef Broth
Cream of Chicken Soup
Beef with Vegetable and Barley Soup
1 Fruit Cocktail
1 Mandarin Oranges, light
15 oz. cans Asparagus
1 can Green Beans
1 can Beets

Breads/Starches
2 loaves Wheat Bread, Pepperidge Farm, light Egg Noodles, regular
2 cans Pringles Fat Free Potato Chips
Angel Hair Spaghetti
English Muffin
English Toasting Bread
1 Box Chicken Stove Top Stuffing Mix
White Rice
White Flour

Miscellaneous
Jam, any flavor
Miracle Whip, regular
Miracle Whip, fat free
Mustard, Grey Poupon
Dill Pickles, medium
Red Wine Vinegar
Pace Salsa
Beef with Vegetable and Barley Soup
Sugar Free Jello
White Wine
Sweet Pickles
Sugar Free Syrup
Fat Free Cooking Spray
Cider Vinegar
Horseradish
Red Wine Vinegar

Oils
Canola Oil
Olive Oil

Nuts/Seeds:
Almonds, slivered

Planned Meals Week 3

Breakfast - 3 Blocks

Eggs with Ham and Salsa

		P	C	F
1	Egg, Whole	6.0	0	5.0
1	Egg White	4.0	0	0
-	Fat Free Cooking Spray	0	0	0
2 T	Pace Salsa	0	3.0	0
1½ slices	Cooked Ham, 96% extra lean	7.5	0	1.5
3 oz.	Milk 2%	3.0	4.3	1.8
3 oz.	Orange Juice	0.8	9.8	0
2 slices	Wheat Bread, Pepperidge Farm, light	4.0	14.0	0.5
1 t	Jam, light	0	3.0	0
½ t	Butter	0	0	1.8
		25.3	34.1	10.6
		3.6	3.7	3.5

Spray a cool skillet with fat free cooking spray. Whisk the egg and egg white and pour into the skillet. Heat the ham in a small skillet. When eggs are almost done move to one side and heat the salsa. (You can omit the salsa and still be in balance.) Toast the bread. Spread one piece with the butter and the other with jam.

Lunch - 3 Blocks

Ham & American Cheese Sandwich (Grapes)

		P	C	F
8 slices	Honey Ham, Deli-Thin 97% lean	13.3	2.6	2.0
2 slices	Wheat Bread, Pepperidge Farm, light	4.0	14.0	0.5
1 T	Miracle Whip, regular	0	2.0	7.0
1	Lettuce Leaf, Romaine	0	0	0
1	American Cheese, fat free	5.0	2.0	0
5	Grapes	0	2.5	0
8	Pringles Fat Free Potato Chips	1.0	6.8	0
		23.3	29.9	9.5
		3.3	3.3	3.1

1/2 of any 2 Block Snack

Dinner - 4 Blocks

Shrimp Scampi for 3   P   C   F

Amount	Ingredient	P	C	F
12 oz.	Shrimp, large, (about 12 each)	72.0	0	4.8
-	Fat Free Cooking Spray	0	0	0
2 T	Butter	0	0	22.0
¼ C	White Wine	0	0	0
5	Garlic Cloves, minced	0	0	0
-	Salt and freshly ground Pepper to taste	0	0	0
1 t	Parsley	0	0	0
3 oz.	Angel Hair Spaghetti	10.0	79.9	1.9
1 oz.	Feta Cheese, crumbled	4.0	1.2	6.0

Mandarin Orange Salad:

Amount	Ingredient	P	C	F
2 C	Romaine Lettuce	6.0	10.0	0
¼ C	Mandarin Oranges, light	0.5	8.0	0
15	Grapes	0	7.5	0
1½ C	Strawberries, diced	1.5	10.5	0
½ T	Almonds, thinly sliced	1.5	1.5	4.0
1 T	Mandarin Orange Salad Dressing	0	3.0	1.1
		95.5	121.6	39.8
		13.6	13.5	13.2
		4.5	4.5	4.4

Mandarin Orange Salad Dressing: Makes 4 Tablespoons.
1 t   Canola Oil
3 T   Mandarin Orange liquid, light
1 t   Red Wine Vinegar
1 t   Cider Vinegar
1 t   Sugar

    Spray a cool skillet with fat a free cooking spray. Add the butter salt, and garlic. Heat over low heat for a few minutes. Raise the heat to medium and add the shrimp. When the shrimp turns pink on one side, turn it over and cook about 2 minutes more. Add the white wine and cook another 30 seconds. Garnish with parsley. Cook spaghetti and add to the skillet, stirring to coat. Heat until warm. Divide shrimp (about 12 each) and spaghetti. Sprinkle with Feta Cheese and freshly ground pepper.
    Prepare the lettuce. Combine salad dressing ingredients, shake well and pour 1 Tablespoon over the lettuce. Mix well. Divide lettuce and put in bowls. Cut grapes in half. Dice the strawberries. Divide the grapes, strawberries and mandarin oranges and place on top of lettuce. Sprinkle almonds on top.
    (You can omit the mandarin oranges and grapes, or the strawberries, and still have a balanced meal.)
    Divide and weigh each meal to assure the meals all weigh the same, within a few tenths of an ounce.
    Sugar Free Flavored Gelatin Dessert that has no PCF's can be eaten anytime you feel like snacking.

1/2 of any 2 Block Snack

Breakfast - 3 Blocks

	Omelet with Ham and Cheese	P	C	F
1	Egg, Whole	6.0	0	5.0
-	Fat Free Cooking Spray	0	0	0
½ slice	Cooked Ham, 96% extra lean	2.5	0	0.5
1 T	Green Pepper, diced	0	0.3	0
1 T	Onion, diced	0	0.3	0
1 slice	American Cheese, fat free	5.0	2.0	0
1 T	Jam, light	0	9.0	0
2 slices	Wheat Bread, Pepperidge Farm, light	4.0	14.0	0.5
½ t	Butter	0	0	1.8
4 oz.	Milk 2%	4.0	5.5	2.5
		21.5	31.1	10.3
		3.0	3.4	3.4

Dice all vegetables and set aside. Spray a cool skillet with fat free cooking spray and heat. Whisk the egg and pour into the skillet. Add the vegetables, ham and cheese on one side of the egg. Fold the other side of the egg over the vegetables. Toast the bread, spread butter on one slice and jam on the other.

Lunch - 3 Blocks

	Tuna Melt	P	C	F
2 oz.	Tuna, water packed	14.9	0	1.0
1 T	Green Onions, chopped	0.1	0.3	0
2 T	Miracle Whip, fat free	0	4.0	0
2 slices	Wheat Bread, Pepperidge Farm, light	4.0	14.0	0.5
1 slices	Swiss Cheese slice, regular	4.0	1.0	5.0
1 t	Butter	0	0	3.6
1	Sweet Pickle, small	0	4.0	0
6	Pringles Fat Free Potato Chips	0.7	6.0	0
2	Strawberry, large	0	1.0	0
		23.7	30.3	10.1
		3.3	3.3	3.3

Spray a cool skillet with fat free cooking spray.
Weigh out 2 ounces of tuna; add the green onions and miracle whip. Blend well. Spread the tuna salad on the bread; spread the butter on the outside of the slices and fry in the skillet until golden brown. Serve with a sweet pickle and Pringles fat free chips. Have the strawberries for a touch of something sweet.

1/2 of any 2 Block Snack

Dinner -4 Blocks

Beef Bourguignon for 4

		P	C	F
16 oz.	Bottom Round, lean	107.5	0	17.2
-	Fat Free Cooking Spray	0	0	0
3 T	Butter	0	0	33.0
2 T	Brandy	0	0	0
6	Pearl Onions	0.6	7.5	0
1 C	Mushrooms, small, whole	0.6	0.9	0.1
2 T	Cornstarch	0	14.0	0
1	Beef Bouillon Cube	0	1.0	0
1 T	Tomato Paste	0.5	2.5	0
½ Can	Beef Broth, condensed	3.7	1.2	0
¾ C	Burgundy Wine	0	0	0
½ C	Dry Sherry	0	0	0
½ C	Ruby Port	0	0	0
1	Bay Leaf	0	0	0
-	Chopped Parsley	0	0	0
1½ C	Egg Noodles, dry	8.0	38.0	2.5
1 C	Romaine Lettuce	3.0	5.0	0
4	Peaches, fresh	0	36.0	0
30	Grapes	0	15.0	0
3 C	Strawberries, diced	3.0	21.0	0
1½ T	Sugar	0	18.0	0
2 T	Mandarin Orange Salad Dressing	0	6.0	2.2
		126.9	162.6	55.0
		18.1	18.0	18.3
		4.5	4.5	4.5

Preheat oven to 350 degrees.

Cut beef into 1½" cubes. Coat with the cornstarch; (shake off excess cornstarch and reserve). Spray a 3-quart Dutch oven (with a tight-fitting lid) with fat free cooking spray. Add 2 tablespoons of butter, and heat. Add beef, a few at a time, until all the pieces are brown.

In a small saucepan, heat 2 T brandy just until vapor rises. Ignite; pour over beef. As flame dies, remove beef cubes to another pan and set aside. Melt 1 tablespoon of butter in Dutch oven, add onions, and cook over low heat, covered, until onions brown slightly, stirring occasionally. Then add the mushrooms, cook, stirring about 3 minutes.

With slotted spoon, remove onions and mushrooms. Remove Dutch oven from heat. Using a wooden spoon, stir in reserved cornstarch, tomato paste and blend well. Stir in Burgundy, sherry, port and beef broth.

Bring wine mixture just to a boil, stirring; remove from heat. Add beef, pepper, bay leaf, onions, mushrooms and remaining brandy; mix well. Place a large sheet of waxed paper over top of the Dutch oven; place lid on top of paper. Bake, covered. Stir occasionally, cook 1 hour, or until beef is tender when pierced with a fork. Pour off liquid collected on paper. Sprinkle with parsley. Serve over egg noodles. Have a fruit salad for dessert.

Divide and weigh each meal to assure the meals all weigh the same, within a few tenths of an ounce.

Sugar Free Flavored Gelatin Dessert that has no PCF's can be eaten anytime you feel like snacking.

1/2 of any 2 Block Snack

Breakfast - 3 Blocks

Eggs Benedict		P	C	F
1	Egg, Whole	6.0	0	5.0
1	Egg, White	4.0	0	0
-	Fat Free Cooking Spray	0	0	0
2 slices	Canadian Bacon, lean	5.0	0.5	0.7
½	English Muffin	2.5	12.5	0.5
3	Potatoes, New, small (6 oz.)	1.9	13.9	0
Hollandaise Sauce:				
1	Egg Yolk	3.0	0	5.0
2 t	Lemon Juice	0	0.8	0
3 T	2% Milk	0	0	0
		22.4	27.7	11.2
		3.2	3.0	3.7

Spray a cool skillet with a fat free cooking spray. Peel potatoes and slice thinly. Fry the potatoes.

Hollandaise Sauce:
 Place egg yolk and milk in top of double boiler. Cook over boiling water, stirring rapidly, until mixture thickens. (Water in the bottom of the double boiler should not touch the top pan.) Remove pan from water and stir rapidly for 2 minutes. Stir in 1 teaspoon of lemon juice at a time. Season with salt and white pepper to taste. Heat again over boiling water, stirring constantly, until thickened. (2 or 3 minutes.) Remove from water at once. If the Hollandaise sauce curdles immediately beat in 1 or 2 t boiling water.

 Place ½ English Muffin on the plate, put on the Canadian Bacon, and then egg. Pour Hollandaise Sauce over top. Serve with fried potatoes.

Lunch - 3 Blocks

Beef with Vegetable & Barley Soup & Tuna Sandwich		P	C	F
½ can	Beef With Vegetable & Barley Soup	6.2	11.2	2.5
2 slices	Wheat Bread, Pepperidge Farm, light	4.0	14.0	0.5
2 oz.	Tuna, albacore, water packed	13.0	0	1.0
2 T	Miracle Whip, fat free	0	4.0	0
1 T	Onions, diced	0.1	0.7	0
1½ t	Butter	0	0	5.4
		23.3	29.9	9.4
		3.3	3.3	3.1

Weigh out 2 ounces of tuna; add the green onions and miracle whip. Blend well. Spread the butter on the bread and add the tuna salad. Heat the soup and serve with the sandwich.

1/2 of any 2 Block Snack

Dinner - 4 Blocks

Teriyaki Chicken with Fruit Salad for 3		P	C	F
12 oz.	Chicken Breasts, skinless, boneless	78.0	0	4.8
6 T	Teriyaki Marinade	6.0	18.0	0
1½ C	White Rice, cooked	6.0	57.0	0
1 C	Broccoli	3.0	6.0	0.5
1½ C	Cauliflower	3.0	7.5	0
3 T	Butter	0	0	33.0

Fruit Salad:

¼ C	Mandarin Oranges, light	0.5	8.0	0
1½ C	Strawberries, sliced	1.5	10.5	0
15	Grapes	0	7.5	0
1 T	Mandarin Orange Salad Dressing	0	3.0	1.1
		98.0	117.5	39.4
		14.0	13.0	13.1
		4.6	4.3	4.3

Mandarin Orange Salad Dressing:
- 1 t — Canola Oil
- 3 T — Mandarin Orange liquid, light
- 1 t — Red Wine Vinegar
- 1 t — Cider Vinegar
- 1 t — Sugar

Teriyaki Marinade:
- ¼ C — Light Brown Sugar, tightly packed
- ½ C — Soy Sauce
- ½ t — Monosodium Glutamate
- ¼ t — Pepper
- 2 T — Lemon Juice
- 1 T — Canola Oil
- 1 T — Ginger Root, grated / or 1 t dry ginger
- 2 — Garlic Clove, minced

    Mix together, add meat, stir to coat and marinate for 2 hours or refrigerate overnight.
    Prepare rice as directed on package but omit the butter.
    Place chicken breasts in a large plastic resealable bag. Make the Teriyaki marinade, pour over the chicken and seal the bag. Turn bag occasionally to make sure the chicken is coated all over. Refrigerate for 3 to 6 hours. You will be making about 1 Cup of Teriyaki mix, but after marinating you will have used only about 2 Tablespoons. Discard leftover marinade. Grill chicken on grill 4 to 5 minutes, turn and grill another 4 to 5 minutes, or until the chicken is no longer pink and the juices run clear.
    (You can omit the Mandarin Oranges, and still be balanced.)
    Divide and weigh each meal to assure the meals all weigh the same, within a few tenths of an ounce.
    Sugar Free Flavored Gelatin Dessert that has no PCF's can be eaten anytime you feel like snacking.

1/2 of any 2 Block Snack

Breakfast - 3 Blocks

French Toast with Ham

		P	C	F
1	Egg, Whole	6.0	0	5.0
1	Egg White	4.0	0	0
-	Fat Free Cooking Spray	0	0	0
2 slices	Wheat Bread, Pepperidge Farm, light	4.0	14.0	0.5
2 T	Syrup, sugar free	0	6.0	0
1 slice	Cooked Ham, 96% extra lean	5.0	0	1.0
½ t	Butter	0	0	1.8
4 oz.	Milk 2%	4.0	5.5	2.5
1½ t	Cinnamon Sugar	0	6.0	0
		23.0	31.5	10.8
		3.2	3.5	3.6

Spray a cool skillet with a fat free cooking spray and heat. Stir egg and egg white, sprinkle a little cinnamon sugar on top of egg mixture and coat the first slice of bread on both sides; place in heated skillet. Sprinkle the remaining cinnamon sugar on top of the eggs and coat the second slice of bread; place in heated skillet. Lightly brown on both sides. Remove bread from skillet and heat the Canadian bacon. You can omit the cinnamon sugar and add another tablespoon of syrup.
Any egg not absorbed by the bread should be fried and served as a side dish.

Lunch - 3 Blocks

Roast Beef Sandwich

		P	C	F
9 slices	Roast Beef, Deli-Thin 98% lean	14.6	2.5	1.0
2 slices	Wheat Bread, Pepperidge Farm, light	4.0	14.0	0.5
2	Lettuce Leaves	0	0	0
1 T	Horseradish	0	0	0
1 T	Miracle Whip, regular	0	2.0	7.0
8	Pringles Fat Free Potato Chips	1.0	6.8	0
1	Dill Pickle, medium	0	1.0	0
		19.6	27.3	8.5
		2.8	2.9	2.8

1/2 of any 2 Block Snack

Dinner - 4 Blocks

Cheesy Fillet of Sole for 3

		P	C	F
10.5 oz.	Fillet of Sole	55.8	0	3.0
1 T	Flour	0.7	5.5	0
½ T	Butter	0	0	5.5
-	Fat Free Cooking Spray	0	0	0
¾ oz.	Gruyere Cheese, grated	6.3	0	6.8
¾ oz.	Monterey Jack Cheese, light, grated	6.7	0.2	4.5
1 C	Milk 2%	8.0	12.0	5.0
2 T	Green Onion tops	0	0	0
1½ C	Broccoli	4.5	9.0	0.7
1½ C	Cauliflower	3.0	7.5	0
1 T	Butter	0	0	11.0
3 slices	Wheat Bread, Pepperidge Farm, light	7.0	22.0	1.0

Dessert:

		P	C	F
3 C	Peaches, fresh (2½" each)	0	27.0	0
1 C	Cool Whip, fat free	0	24.0	0
1 t	Sugar	0	4.0	0
		92.0	111.2	37.5
		13.1	12.3	12.5
		4.3	4.1	4.1

Thaw frozen fish in milk, or if it's fresh, soak in the milk until ready to cook. Discard the left over milk. Spray a cool skillet with a fat free cooking spray. Heat skillet. Coat the fish with flour and fry until it flakes easily.

Melt cheese and whisk with milk until smooth, and stir in the green onions. When fish is done, place on the plates, and cover with the cheese sauce.

Steam vegetables and melt the butter over the top. Serve fresh peaches and fat free whipped topping for dessert.

(You can substitute 3 medium Apples, or 2 Cups of Fruit Cocktail, water packed instead of the peaches, Cool Whip, (fat free) and sugar. Or try another substitution.)

Divide and weigh each meal to assure the meals all weigh the same, within a few tenths of an ounce.

Sugar Free Flavored Gelatin Dessert that has no PCF's can be eaten anytime you feel like snacking.

1/2 of any 2 Block Snack

Breakfast - 3 Blocks

	Omelet with Ham and Cheese	P	C	F
1	Egg, Whole	6.0	0	5.0
-	Fat Free Cooking Spray	0	0	0
½ slice	Cooked Ham, 96% extra lean	2.5	0	0.5
1 T	Green Pepper, diced	0	0.3	0
1 T	Onion, diced	0	0.3	0
1 slice	American Cheese, fat free	5.0	2.0	0
1 T	Jam, light	0	9.0	0
2 slices	Wheat Bread, Pepperidge Farm, light	4.0	14.0	0.5
½ t	Butter	0	0	1.8
4 oz.	Milk 2%	4.0	5.5	2.5
		21.5	31.1	10.3
		3.0	3.4	3.4

Spray a cool skillet with fat free cooking spray. Brown the ham, green pepper and onions. Remove from skillet; Whisk the egg and fry. When the egg is almost done, add the cooked vegetables and ham, tear up the cheese and place on top of the vegetables. Spread one piece of toast with butter and the other with jam.

Lunch - 3 Blocks

	Tuna Sandwich	P	C	F
2.5 oz.	Tuna, Albacore, water packed	18.7	0	1.3
2 slices	Wheat Bread, Pepperidge Farm, light	4.0	14.0	0.5
2 T	Onion, diced	0	1.4	0.2
2	Lettuce Leaves	0	0	0
1 T	Miracle Whip, regular	0	2.0	7.0
1	Sweet Pickle, small	0	4.0	0
8	Pringles Fat Free Potato Chips	1.0	6.8	0
		23.7	28.2	9.3
		3.3	3.1	3.1

(A 9 oz. can of tuna makes 3 sandwiches. After draining, there is 7.5 oz of tuna.)

Weigh the tuna, stir in the diced onion and Miracle Whip. Place the tuna mixture on the bread and add the lettuce. Salt and pepper to taste. Serve with a sweet pickle and chips.

1/2 of any 2 Block Snack

Dinner - 4 Blocks

Pork Loin Chops with Cole Slaw for 3

		P	C	F
10.5 oz.	Pork Loin Chops (3.5 oz. each)	65.1	0	21.0
-	Fat Free Cooking Spray	0	0	0
-	Salt and Pepper to taste	0	0	0
1 Can	Asparagus Spears	7.0	7.0	0
1½ C	Cauliflower	3.0	7.5	0
1 Can	Beets	3.0	21.0	0
1½ T	Butter	0	0	16.5
Cole Slaw:				
2 C	Cabbage, shredded	2.0	6.6	0
4 T	Miracle Whip, fat free	0	8.0	0
1 T	Milk 2%	0.5	0.7	0.3
1 t	Cider Vinegar	0	0	0
2 t	Sugar	0	8.0	0
1 can	Fruit Cocktail, in juice	0	49.0	0
		80.6	107.8	37.8
		11.5	11.9	12.6
		3.8	3.9	4.2

Mix together, miracle whip, milk, cider vinegar and sugar. Shred cabbage. Pour mixture over shredded cabbage and chill.

Trim all visible fat from the pork chops before weighing. Spray a cool skillet with fat free cooking spray and heat. Fry pork chops until the meat is no longer pink.

Heat the beets and asparagus. Steam the cauliflower. Melt ½ Tablespoon of the butter over each vegetable.

Divide the fruit cocktail and serve as dessert. (You can omit the fruit cocktail and add 5 Cups of diced watermelon and still be in balance. Or try another substitution.)

Divide and weigh each meal to assure the meals all weigh the same, within a few tenths of an ounce.

Sugar Free Flavored Gelatin Dessert that has no PCF's can be eaten anytime you feel like snacking.

1/2 of any 2 Block Snack

Breakfast - 2 Blocks

Poached Eggs with English Toasting Bread		P	C	F
1	Egg, Poached	6.0	0	5.0
-	Fat Free Cooking Spray	0	0	0
2 slices	Canadian bacon, lean	5.5	0	0.7
1 slice	English Toasting Bread	3.0	14.0	1.0
2 t	Jam, light	0	6.0	0
2 oz.	Milk 2%	2.0	2.7	1.2
		16.5	22.7	7.9
		2.3	2.5	2.6

Spray a small, cool skillet with fat free cooking spray, add enough water to cover egg. Cook over medium heat until done. While the egg is poaching, heat the bacon. Serve with toast and jam.

Lunch - 3 Blocks

Ham & American Cheese Sandwich (Grapes)		P	C	F
8 slices	Honey Ham, Deli-Thin 97% lean	13.3	2.6	2.0
2 slices	Wheat Bread, Pepperidge Farm, light	4.0	14.0	0.5
1 T	Miracle Whip, regular	0	2.0	7.0
1	Lettuce Leaf, Romaine	0	0	0
1	American Cheese, fat free	5.0	2.0	0
5	Grapes	0	2.5	0
8	Pringles Fat Free Potato Chips	1.0	6.8	0
		23.3	29.9	9.5
		3.3	3.3	3.1

1/2 of any 2 Block Snack

Dinner - 5 Blocks

Beef Stroganoff for 3

		P	C	F
10 oz.	Top Sirloin Steak	86.0	0	19.2
2 C	Onions, diced	3.6	22.4	0.4
-	Fat Free Cooking Spray	0	0	0
2 T	Butter	0	0	22.0
-	Salt and Pepper to taste	0	0	0
4.5 oz. can	Mushrooms, with juice	1.0	2.0	0
1	Beef Bouillon Cube	0	1.0	0
2 T	Cornstarch	0	14.0	0
1½ C	Water	0	0	0
½ C	Sour Cream, fat free	8.0	16.0	0
3 oz.	Egg Noodles, 2 C dry	8.0	38.0	2.4

Mandarin Orange Salad:

2 C	Romaine Lettuce	6.0	10.0	0
27	Grapes	0	12.5	0
1½ C	Strawberries, sliced	1.5	10.5	0
1 C	Mandarin Oranges, light	1.0	16.0	0
1 T	Mandarin Orange Salad Dressing	0	3.0	1.1
		115.1	145.4	45.1
		16.4	16.1	15.0
		5.4	5.3	5.0

Mandarin Orange Salad Dressing: (Makes 4 Tablespoons.)

1 t	Canola Oil
3 T	Mandarin Orange liquid, light
1 t	Red Wine Vinegar
1 t	Cider Vinegar
1 t	Sugar

    Cook noodles according to the package directions and set aside. (Run hot water over the noodles to reheat when ready to serve.)

    Cut Steak into thin strips. Spray a cool skillet with a fat free cooking spray. Add butter and heat. Add meat strips and onions and brown. (About 10 minutes.) Add beef bouillon cube, salt, pepper, ½ Cup of water and liquid from the canned mushrooms. Bring to a boil, reduce heat to low, cover and simmer about ½ hour, or until meat is fork tender, adding water as needed to keep meat from burning. Add the mushrooms and heat. Remove beef mixture to a warm plate. Keep warm. Stir the cornstarch and 1½ Cups of water together and gradually add to the skillet. Cook over medium heat until the sauce thickens. Stir in the sour cream. Heat thoroughly but do not boil. Return beef to the skillet and stir, making sure to coat beef completely. Divide the noodles and beef. Spoon the beef mixture over the noodles and serve.

    Combine salad dressing ingredients, shake well and pour 1 Tablespoons over the lettuce. Mix well, divide and place in bowls. Cut Grapes in half. Divide mandarin oranges, strawberries and grapes. Place on top of the lettuce. (You can omit the strawberries, grapes or mandarin oranges and still have a balanced meal.)

    Divide and weigh each meal to assure the meals all weigh the same, within a few tenths of an ounce.

    Sugar Free Flavored Gelatin Dessert that has no PCF's can be eaten anytime you feel like snacking.

1/2 of any 2 Block Snack

Breakfast - 4 Blocks

French Toast

		P	C	F
1	Egg, Whole	6.0	0	5.0
2	Egg Whites	8.0	0	0
-	Fat Free Cooking Spray	0	0	0
2 slices	Wheat Bread, Pepperidge Farm, light	4.0	14.0	0.5
2 T	Syrup, sugar free	0	6.0	0
1 slice	Cooked Ham, 96% extra lean	5.0	0	1.0
1 t	Butter	0	0	3.6
4 oz.	Milk 2%	4.0	5.5	2.5
1 T	Cinnamon Sugar	0	12.0	0
		27.0	37.5	12.6
		3.8	4.1	4.2

Spray a cool skillet with fat free cooking spray and heat. Stir egg and egg whites, sprinkle a little cinnamon sugar on top of egg mixture and coat the first slice of bread on both sides; place in heated skillet. Sprinkle the remaining cinnamon sugar on top of the eggs and coat the second slice of bread; place in heated skillet. Lightly brown on both sides. Remove bread from skillet and heat the Canadian bacon. You can omit the cinnamon sugar and add another tablespoon of syrup. Any egg not absorbed by the bread should be fried and served as a side dish.

Lunch - 2 Blocks

Grilled Ham and Cheese Sandwich

		P	C	F
2 slices	Wheat Bread, Pepperidge Farm, light	4.0	14.0	0.5
2 slices	American Cheese, reduced fat	8.0	4.0	6.0
½ T	Miracle Whip, fat free	0	1.0	0
1 slice	Cooked Ham, 96% extra lean	5.0	0	1.0
4	Pringles Fat Free Potato Chips	0.5	3.4	0
-	Salt and Pepper to taste	0	0	0
		17.5	22.4	7.5
		2.5	2.5	2.5

Spray a skillet with fat free cooking spray. Prepare the sandwich and sprinkle with salt and pepper. Spread butter on each slice of bread and grill sandwich until golden brown. Serve with chips on the side.

1/2 of any 2 Block Snack

Dinner - 4 Blocks

Chicken & Stuffing Bake for 3		P	C	F
12 oz.	Chicken Breasts, skinless, boneless	78.0	0	4.8
-	Fat Free Cooking Spray	0	0	0
2 C	Stove Top Chicken Stuffing Mix	12.0	76.0	4.0
2 T	Butter	0	0	22.0
½ Can	Cream of Chicken Soup	3.2	7.2	6.4
¼ C	Milk 2%	2.0	3.0	1.2
½ t	Parsley, dried	0	0	0
1 Can	Green Beans	1.0	13.5	0
Mandarin Orange Salad:				
1 C	Romaine Lettuce	3.0	5.0	0
¼ C	Mandarin Oranges, light	0.5	8.0	0
1 C	Strawberries, sliced	1.0	7.0	0
1 T	Mandarin Orange Salad Dressing	0	3.0	1.1
		100.7	122.7	39.5
		14.3	13.6	13.1
		4.7	4.5	4.3

Mandarin Orange Salad Dressing: Makes 4 Tablespoons
- 1 t — Canola Oil
- 3 T — Mandarin Orange liquid, light
- 1 t — Red Wine Vinegar
- 1 t — Cider Vinegar
- 1 t — Sugar

Pre-heat the oven to 400 degrees. Spray a cool skillet with fat free cooking spray and brown the chicken. Make the stuffing according to the directions on the box. Spoon 2 Cups of the stuffing mixture down the center of a 3-quart casserole dish. Arrange chicken breasts on both sides of stuffing. Sprinkle chicken with paprika, salt and pepper. Mix soup, milk and parsley. Pour over chicken. Bake at 400 degrees for 30 minutes, or until chicken is no longer pink and juice runs clear. Serve with Green beans and salad.

Combine salad dressing ingredients, shake well and pour 1 Tablespoon over the lettuce, mix well, divide and place in bowls. Divide mandarin oranges and strawberries, place on top of lettuce.

(You can omit the strawberries and substitute 10 grapes and still have a balanced meal.)

Divide and weigh each meal to assure the meals all weigh the same, within a few tenths of an ounce.

Sugar Free Flavored Gelatin Dessert that has no PCF's can be eaten anytime you feel like snacking.

1/2 of any 2 Block Snack

Weight and Measurements
Results Week 3

Name　　　_____
Weight　_____
Arm　　　_____
Chest　　_____
Waist　　_____
Hips　　　_____
Thigh　　_____

Name　　　_____
Weight　_____
Arm　　　_____
Chest　　_____
Waist　　_____
Hips　　　_____
Thigh　　_____

Name　　　_____
Weight　_____
Arm　　　_____
Chest　　_____
Waist　　_____
Hips　　　_____
Thigh　　_____

Name　　　_____
Weight　_____
Arm　　　_____
Chest　　_____
Waist　　_____
Hips　　　_____
Thigh　　_____

Grocery List
Week 4

Fresh Fruits and Vegetables
3 Tangerines
Grapes
3 Lemon
5 C Strawberries
2 Green Peppers
2 Romaine Lettuce (or mixed greens)
3 Tomato
Carrots
Snow Peas
Cauliflower
Garlic Cloves
Green Onions
Onions
Red Potatoes
Tarragon, fresh
3 Corn on the Cob or
11 oz can of Corn

Meats
34 oz Ground Beef, 93%
24 oz. Chicken Breasts, skinless, boneless
12 oz. Pork Tenderloin
12 oz Orange Roughy (or any white fish)
12 oz Halibut (or any white fish)
Tuna, Albacore, water-packed, canned
Breakfast Sausage 97% (fat free made with pork and turkey)

Lunch Meats
Canadian Bacon, lean
Cooked Ham, 96%
Honey Ham, Deli-Thin, 97% lean
Corned Beef Deli-Thin, lean
Pastrami 98% lean

Dairy
1 Doz. Eggs
Butter
2 % Milk
American Cheese, fat free, slices
Swiss Cheese slices, fat free
Parmesan Cheese, regular
2 Whipped Topping, fat free
Orange Juice
Cheddar Cheese, fat free
Cheddar Cheese, regular

Canned Fruits/Vegetables
1-28 oz. Whole Tomatoes
3-15 oz. Tomato Sauce
15 oz Italian Tomatoes
3 Mandarin Oranges, light
15 oz. cans Asparagus
1 can Green Beans
2-11 oz can Corn
Peas, frozen

Breads/Starches
2 loaves Wheat Bread, Pepperidge Farm, light
Oatmeal
Lasagna Noodles
Angel Food Cake Mix
Smart Start Cereal
English Toasting Bread
Pringles Fat Free Potato Chips
White Rice

Nuts/Seeds
Almonds slivered

Miscellaneous
Miracle Whip fat free
Miracle Whip regular
Jam, any flavor

Sweet Pickles, small
Dill Pickles, medium
Sweet Pickle Relish
Fat free Cooking Spray
Worcestershire Sauce
Raisins, dark
Heinz Ketchup
Brown Sugar
Red Wine
Pace Salsa
Cider Vinegar
Red Wine Vinegar
White Wine Vinegar
Sugar Free Jello
Mustard
Vegetarian Vegetable Soup
Horseradish

Oils:
Olive Oil
Canola Oil

Spices:
Parsley Flakes
Bay Leaf
Garlic, Granulated
Cinnamon/Sugar

Planned Meals Week 4

Breakfast - 3 Blocks

Sausage and Egg with Orange Juice

		P	C	F
1	Egg, Whole	6.0	0	5.0
-	Fat Free Cooking Spray	0	0	0
2	Breakfast Sausage, 97% fat free	0	0	0
-	(Made with pork and turkey)	7.0	3.0	1.5
1 slice	Wheat Bread, Pepperidge Farm, light	1.0	7.0	0
3 oz.	Milk 2%	3.0	1.8	1.8
4 oz.	Orange Juice	1.0	13.0	0
½ t	Butter	0	0	1.8
		19.0	28.5	10.1
		2.7	3.1	3.3

Spray a cool skillet with fat free cooking spray and fry the egg. Heat the sausage in a small skillet. Spread the butter on the toast and serve with milk and orange juice.

Lunch - 3 Blocks

Tuna Sandwich

		P	C	F
2.5 oz.	Tuna, Albacore, water packed	18.7	0	1.3
2 slices	Wheat Bread, Pepperidge Farm, light	4.0	14.0	0.5
2 T	Onion, diced	0	1.4	0.2
2	Lettuce Leaves	0	0	0
1 T	Miracle Whip, regular	0	2.0	7.0
1	Sweet Pickle, small	0	4.0	0
8	Pringles Fat Free Potato Chips	1.0	6.8	0
		23.7	28.2	9.3
		3.3	3.1	3.1

Weigh the tuna and mix in the diced onions and Miracle Whip together. Salt and pepper to taste. Add the lettuce. Serve with a sweet pickle and chips.

       (9-oz. can of tuna makes 3 sandwiches)
       (After draining, there is 7.5 oz of tuna.)

1/2 of any 2 Block Snack

Dinner - 4 Blocks

Grilled Halibut for 3

		P	C	F
12 oz.	Halibut Fillets (or any other white fish)	48.0	0	3.0
-	Fat Free Cooking Spray	0	0	0
1 T	Butter	0	0	11.0
3 T	Heinz Ketchup	0	12.0	0
11 oz.	Corn (canned)	8.0	40.0	2.0
1 Can	Asparagus (15 oz.)	7.0	7.0	0
1 T	Butter	0	0	11.0
24 oz.	Milk, 2% (8 oz. each)	24.0	33.0	15.0

Mandarin Orange Salad:

1 C	Romaine Lettuce	3.0	5.0	0
20	Grapes	0	10.0	0
1 C	Strawberries, sliced	1.0	7.0	0
1 t	Sugar	0	4.0	0
1 T	Mandarin Orange Salad Dressing	0	3.0	1.1
		91.0	121.0	41.1
		13.0	13.4	13.7
		4.3	4.4	4.5

Mandarin Orange Salad Dressing: Makes 4 Tablespoons.

1 t	Canola Oil
3 T	Mandarin Orange liquid, light
1 t	Red Wine Vinegar
1 t	Cider Vinegar
1 t	Sugar

Thaw fish in a little milk until ready to cook. Discard the left over milk. Sprinkle fish with salt and pepper and fry or grill until the fish flakes. While the fish is grilling, heat the vegetables and put ½ T of butter on each. Divide by 3 and serve.

You can substitute 5 T of fat free Miracle Whip for the 3 Tablespoons of ketchup (or a combination) and still be balanced.

Combine salad dressing ingredients, shake well and pour 1 Tablespoon of dressing over the lettuce, mix well, divide and place in bowls. Cut Grapes in half. Chop strawberries. Divide strawberries and grapes, and place on top of lettuce.

(You can omit strawberries and grapes and still have a balanced meal.) OR (You can omit Miracle Whip and ketchup and still be balanced.)

Divide and weigh each meal to assure the meals all weigh the same, within a few tenths of an ounce.
Sugar Free Jello has no PCF's and can be eaten anytime you feel like snacking.

1/2 of any 2 Block Snack

Breakfast - 4 Blocks

Eggs with Toast and Ham

		P	C	F
1	Egg, Whole	6.0	0	5.0
1	Egg White	4.0	0	0
-	Fat Free Cooking Spray	0	0	0
2 slices	Wheat Toast, Pepperidge Farm, light	4.0	14.0	0.5
3 oz.	Milk 2%	3.0	4.5	1.2
4 oz.	Orange Juice	1.0	13.0	0
2 t	Jam, light	0	6.0	0
1 t	Butter	0	0	3.6
2 slices	Cooked Ham, 96% extra lean	10.0	0	2.0
		28.0	37.5	12.3
		4.0	4.1	4.1

Spray a cool skillet with fat free cooking spray. Put the egg and egg white into the skillet and fry, being careful not to break the yolk. Heat the ham. Toast the bread and spread one piece with butter and the other with jam.

Lunch - 2 Blocks

Beef with Vegetable & Barley Soup

		P	C	F
½ can	Beef With Vegetable & Barley	6.2	13.7	2.5
1	Hard Boiled Egg	6.0	0	5.0
½ oz.	Cheddar Cheese, reduced fat	4.0	0.5	0
1	Tangerine	0	9.0	0
		16.2	23.2	7.5
		2.3	2.5	2.5

Place the egg in a pan of cold water. Bring to a boil, cover and remove from heat. Let sit for 20 minutes and shell the egg. Heat the soup. Serve with a small hunk of cheese and a tangerine.

1/2 of any 2 Block Snack

Dinner - 4 Blocks

Meat Loaf for 3

		P	C	F
14 oz.	Ground Beef, 93% lean	73.5	0	21.0
2 slices	Wheat Bread, light	4.0	14.0	0.5
½ C	Onions, diced	0.4	2.8	0
¼ C	Green Pepper, diced	0.1	1.4	0
1	Egg	4.0	0	5.0
-	Non-Stick Spray	0	0	0
9 T	Heinz Ketchup	0	36.0	0
1½ C	Cauliflower	3.0	7.5	0
1 Can	Asparagus	7.0	7.0	0
1½ T	Butter	0	0	16.5

Dessert:

3 C	Strawberries, sliced	3.0	21.0	0
¾ C	Cool Whip, fat free	0	18.0	0
1 T	Sugar	0	12.0	0
		95.0	119.7	43.0
		13.5	13.3	14.3
		4.5	4.4	4.7

Place ground beef in a large bowl. Mix in the bread crumbs, onions, green pepper, and egg. Blend well and shape in a loaf pan. Salt and Pepper to taste. Bake in the oven at 350 degree for about 1 hour, or until the meatloaf is no longer pink.

Steam cauliflower. Heat asparagus. Divide butter in half and melt over each of the vegetables.

(You can omit the strawberries and sugar with Cool Whip, fat free, substitute 3 slices of Wheat Bread, Pepperidge Farm, light, minus the butter, and 6 more tablespoons of ketchup. You will still be eating a 4-block meal. Or you can substitute something else.)

Divide and weigh each meal to assure the meals all weigh the same, within a few tenths of an ounce.

Sugar Free Flavored Gelatin Dessert that has no PCF's can be eaten anytime you feel like snacking.

1/2 of any 2 Block Snack

Breakfast - 3 Blocks

Sausage and Eggs with Potatoes and Strawberries

		P	C	F
1	Egg, Whole	6.0	0	5.0
1	Egg White	4.0	0	0
-	Fat Free Cooking Spray	0	0	0
2	Potato, small red (4 oz.)	1.2	9.2	0
1 med.	Tomato, slices	1.0	6.0	0
1	Breakfast Sausage, 97% fat free	0	0	0
-	(Made with pork and turkey)	3.5	1.5	0.7
1 slice	Wheat Toast, Pepperidge Farm, light	2.0	7.0	0
3 oz.	Milk 2%	3.0	1.8	1.8
½ C	Strawberries	0.5	3.5	0
½ t	Butter	0	0	1.8
		21.2	29.0	9.3
		3.0	3.2	3.1

Peel potatoes and slice in thin slices. Spray a cool skillet with fat free cooking spray and fry the potatoes until tender and brown. Spray another skillet and fry the egg and egg white. Heat the sausage.

Lunch - 3 Blocks

Hot Pastrami

		P	C	F
6 slices	Pastrami, 98% Deli Select	11.0	1.0	1.0
2 slices	Rye Bread	4.0	22.0	2.0
1½ slices	Swiss Cheese, fat free	7.5	4.5	0
2 T	Mustard, Grey Poupon	0	0	0
2 slices	Onion, thin sliced	0	0	0
2 t	Butter	0	0	7.0
1	Dill Pickle, medium	0	1.0	0
		22.5	28.5	10.0
		3.2	3.1	3.3

Spray a cool skillet with fat free cooking spray. Make the sandwich; spread the butter on the outside of the bread and fry until golden brown. Serve with the dill pickle.

1/2 of any 2 Block Snack

Dinner - 4 Blocks

Orange Chicken with Green Grapes for 3

		P	C	F
12 oz.	Chicken Breasts, skinless, boneless	78.0	0	4.8
-	Fat Free Cooking Spray	0	0	0
1 T	Butter	0	0	11.0
-	Salt and Pepper to taste	0	0	0
¼ t	Paprika	0	0	0
½ C	Orange Juice	2.0	26.0	0
1 T	Green Onions, chopped	0	0	0
1	Chicken Bouillon Cube	0	1.0	0
1 T	Cornstarch	0	7.0	0
30	Green Grapes, seedless, halved	0	15.0	0
11 oz.	Corn (canned)	8.0	40.0	2.0
1 T	Butter	0	0	11.0
8	Red Potatoes, small (16 oz. peeled)	4.0	28.0	0
¼ C	Cheddar Cheese, fat free, grated	8.0	1.0	1.5
2 T	Green Onions, chopped	0	0.6	0
1 T	Butter	0	0	11.0
		100.0	118.6	41.3
		14.2	13.1	13.1
		4.7	4.3	4.3

Spray a cool skillet with fat free cooking spray and brown chicken on all sides.

Preheat oven to 350 degrees. Arrange chicken in a 13 x 9 x 2 Baking pan. Season with salt, pepper and paprika.

In a small bowl mix together orange juice, green onions, and bouillon cube. Pour mixture over chicken and bake until the chicken is no longer pink and the juices run clear. Remove chicken and place on a platter and keep warm.

Dissolved the cornstarch in 1 T of water and stir into pan drippings and bring to a boil. Cook until thick and bubbly, stirring constantly. Add grapes and cook until hot.

While chicken is cooking, peel potatoes, dice and steam. Mash the potatoes; stir in cheddar cheese, green onions, and 1 Tablespoon of butter. Keep warm until ready to serve. Heat the corn and melt 1 T of butter over the top before serving.

Divide and weigh each meal to assure the meals all weigh the same, within a few tenths of an ounce.

Sugar Free Jello has no PCF's and can be eaten anytime you feel like snacking.

1/2 of any 2 Block Snack

Breakfast - 2 Blocks

Shredded Wheat   P   C   F

		P	C	F
1	Shredded Wheat Biscuit	2.5	16.5	1.5
3 oz.	Milk 2%	3.0	4.5	1.8
½ t	Sugar	0	2.0	0
1	Egg, Whole	6.0	0	5.0
-	Fat Free Cooking Spray	0	0	0
1 slice	American Cheese, fat free	5.0	2.0	0
		15.5	25.0	8.3
		2.4	2.7	2.7

Spray a cool skillet with fat free cooking spray; add the egg and fry. Melt the cheese on the egg and serve with the cereal.

Lunch - 4 Blocks

Reuben Sandwich

		P	C	F
8 slices	Corned Beef, Healthy Deli, lean	15.2	1.8	2.6
2 slices	Pepperidge Farm Pumpernickel Bread	6.0	23.6	2.0
1 slice	Swiss Cheese, fat free	5.0	3.0	0
¼ C	Sauerkraut	0	2.0	0
2 T	Thousand Island Dressing, fat free	0	6.0	0
1 T	Miracle Whip, fat free	0	2.0	0
2 t	Butter	0	0	7.3
1	Dill Pickle, medium	0	1.0	0
		26.2	39.4	11.9
		3.7	4.3	3.9

Make the sandwich. Mix the Miracle Whip and Thousand Island dressing together and spread on the bread. Add the rest of the ingredients. Spread the butter on the outside of the bread and fry in a skillet until golden brown. Serve with a dill pickle or omit the pickle and still be balanced.

1/2 of any 2 Block Snack

Dinner - 4 Blocks

	Stuffed Orange Roughy for 3	P	C	F
12 oz.	Orange Roughy (or any other white fish)	64.0	0	4.0
-	Fat Free Cooking Spray	0	0	0
2 T	Butter	0	0	22.0
1 T	Lemon juice	0	1.0	0
-	Salt & Pepper to taste	0	0	0
Rice Stuffing:				
1 C	*Rice, cooked	4.0	38.0	0
½ C	Carrots, diced small	1.0	11.5	0
½ C	Peas, frozen	3.7	6.0	0.2
2 T	Green Onion tops, sliced	0.2	0.6	0
4	Lemon Slices, thin sliced	0	1.0	0
1 can	Asparagus	7.0	7.0	0
1 T	Butter	0	0	11.0
Mandarin Orange Salad:				
3 C	Romaine Lettuce	9.0	15.0	0
¼ C	Mandarin Oranges, light	0.5	8.0	0
15	Grapes	0	7.5	0
2 T	Mandarin Orange Salad Dressing	0	6.0	2.2
		89.4	101.6	39.4
		12.7	11.2	13.1
		4.2	3.7	4.3

Mandarin Orange Salad Dressing: Makes 4 Tablespoons.
1 t	Canola Oil
3 T	Mandarin Orange liquid, light
1 t	Red Wine Vinegar
1 t	Cider Vinegar
1 t	Sugar

Prepare rice as directed on package but omit the butter. About 5 minutes before the rice is done, add the diced carrots, peas and green onion tops. Continue cooking until vegetables are tender.

Thaw fish in milk. Discard the left over milk. Spray a cool skillet with fat free cooking spray and add the 2 T butter. Heat skillet, sprinkle the fish with salt and pepper, squeeze the lemon juice evenly over fish, and fry fish until it flakes, (7 to 10 min)

Combine salad dressing ingredients, shake well and pour 2 Tablespoons of dressing over the lettuce, mix well, divide and place in bowls. Cut grapes in half. Divide mandarin oranges and grapes and place on top of lettuce.

Divide and weigh each meal to assure the meals all weigh the same, within a few tenths of an ounce. Sugar Free Flavored Gelatin Dessert that has no PCF's can be eaten anytime you want a snack.

1/2 of any 2 Block Snack

Breakfast - 3 Blocks

Omelet with Ham and Cheese

		P	C	F
1	Egg, Whole	6.0	0	5.0
-	Fat Free Cooking Spray	0	0	0
½ slice	Cooked Ham, 96% extra lean	2.5	0	0.5
1 T	Green Pepper, diced	0	0.3	0
1 T	Onion, diced	0	0.3	0
1 slice	American Cheese, fat free	5.0	2.0	0
1 T	Jam, light	0	9.0	0
2 slices	Wheat Toast, Pepperidge Farm, light	4.0	14.0	0.5
½ t	Butter	0	0	1.8
4 oz.	Milk 2%	4.0	5.5	2.5
		21.5	31.1	10.3
		3.0	3.4	3.4

Spray a cool skillet with fat free cooking spray. Brown the ham, green pepper and onions in a small skillet. Whisk the egg and pour into another skillet. When the egg is almost done, add the cooked ham and vegetables. Tear up the cheese and lay over top of vegetables. Spread one piece of toast with butter and the other with jam.

Lunch - 3 Blocks

Ham & Swiss Cheese Sandwich

		P	C	F
8 slices	Honey Ham, Deli-Thin 97% lean	13.3	2.6	2.0
2 slices	Wheat Bread, Pepperidge Farm, light	4.0	14.0	0.5
1 T	Miracle Whip, regular	0	2.0	7.0
1	Lettuce Leaf, Romaine	0	0	0
1 slice	Swiss Cheese, fat free	5.0	3.0	0
2 t	Horseradish	0	2.0	0
6	Pringles Fat Free Potato Chips	0.7	6.0	0
		22.7	29.6	9.5
		3.2	3.2	3.1

1/2 of any 2 Block Snack

Dinner - 4 Blocks

Pork Chops with Stuffing and for 3

		P	C	F
12 oz.	Pork Chops	68.0	0	20.0
-	Fat Free Cooking Spray	0	0	0
2 C	Stove Top Pork Chop Stuffing Mix	12.0	76.0	1.2
1 Can	Asparagus	7.0	7.0	0
1½ T	Butter	0	0	16.5
2 C	Romaine Lettuce	6.0	10.0	0
¼ C	Mandarin Oranges, light	0.5	8.0	0
10	Grapes	0	5.0	0
1 C	Strawberries, sliced	1.0	7.0	0
2 T	Mandarin Orange Salad Dressing	0	6.0	2.2
		94.5	119.0	39.9
		13.5	13.2	13.3
		4.5	4.4	4.4

Mandarin Orange Salad Dressing: Makes 4 Tablespoons.
1 t	Canola Oil
3 T	Mandarin Orange liquid, light
1 t	Red Wine Vinegar
1 t	Cider Vinegar
1 t	Sugar

Spray a cool skillet with fat free cooking spray and fry pork chops until they are no longer pink. Make the Stove Top Stuffing, but omit the butter. Use only 2 cups of the stuffing. Heat the asparagus and melt the butter over it.

(You can omit the asparagus, use 1½ Cups of dressing and an 11-oz. can of corn, and the meal will still be balanced.)

Combine salad dressing ingredients, shake well and pour 2 Tablespoons of dressing over the lettuce, mix well, divide and place in bowls. Cut grapes in half. Chop strawberries. Divide mandarin oranges grapes and strawberries and place on top of lettuce.

(You can omit the grapes or strawberries and still have a balanced meal.)
Divide and weigh each meal to assure the meals all weigh the same, within a few tenths of an ounce.

Sugar Free Flavored Gelatin Dessert that has no PCF's can be eaten anytime you want a snack.

1/2 of any 2 Block Snack

Breakfast - 3 Block

Sausage and Eggs with Potatoes and Jam		P	C	F
1	Egg, Whole	6.0	0	5.0
1	Egg White	4.0	0	0
-	Fat Free Cooking Spray	0	0	0
2	Potato, small red (4 oz.)	1.2	9.2	0
½ med.	Tomato, slices	0.5	3.0	0
2	Breakfast Sausage, 97% fat free	0	0	0
-	(Made with pork and turkey)	7.0	3.0	1.5
1 slice	Wheat Toast, Pepperidge Farm, light	2.0	7.0	0
3 oz.	Milk 2%	3.0	1.8	1.8
2 t	Jam, light	0	6.0	0
½ t	Butter	0	0	1.8
		23.7	30.0	10.1
		3.3	3.3	3.3

Spray a skillet with fat free cooking spray and scramble eggs, spray another cool skillet with non-stick spray and fry the potatoes. Cook the sausage according to the package directions. Spread butter on 1 slice of toast, and jam on the other.

Lunch - 3 Blocks

Tuna Melt		P	C	F
2 oz.	Tuna, water packed	14.9	0	1.0
1 T	Green Onions, chopped	0.1	0.3	0
2 T	Miracle Whip, fat free	0	4.0	0
2 slices	Wheat Bread, Pepperidge Farm, light	4.0	14.0	0.5
1 slices	Swiss Cheese slice, regular	4.0	1.0	5.0
1 t	Butter	0	0	3.6
-	Fat Free Cooking Spray	0	0	0
1	Sweet Pickle, small	0	4.0	0
6	Pringles Fat Free Potato Chips	0.7	6.0	0
2	Strawberry, large	0	1.0	0
		23.7	30.3	10.1
		3.3	3.3	3.3

Spray a cool skillet with fat free cooking spray. Make the sandwich, spread the butter on the outside of each slice of bread and grill sandwich until golden brown. Serve with a sweet pickle, strawberries and chips.

1/2 of any 2 Block Snack

Dinner - 4 Blocks

Spaghetti for 6

		P	C	F
20 oz.	Ground Beef, 93%	105.0	0	30.0
½ C	Onions, diced	0.9	5.6	0.1
28 oz.	Whole Tomatoes	7.0	21.0	0
45 oz.	Tomato Sauce	21.0	42.0	0
1 T	Brown Sugar	0	12.0	0
2 T	Oregano	0	0	0
¼ C	Parsley Flakes	0	0	0
½ t	Garlic, granulated	0	0	0
1/8 t	Thyme	0	0	0
1	Bay Leaf	0	0	0
6 oz.	Angel Hair Spaghetti	21.0	120.0	3.0
6 T	Parmesan Cheese, regular, grated	18.0	0	13.8
6 slices	Wheat Bread, Pepperidge Farm, light	14.0	44.0	2.0
½ t	Garlic, granulated	0	0	0
3 T	Butter	0	0	33.0
		186.9	244.6	81.9
		26.7	27.1	27.3
		4.4	4.5	4.5

Makes about ¾ C each serving.

Brown meat and onions in skillet. Add the next 8 ingredients, and simmer about 2 hours, or until sauce is thick. Cook the 6-oz. spaghetti. (Use spices to suit your own taste.)

Divide and weigh the cooked spaghetti and place on 6 plates. Discard Bay Leaf. Pour ¾ C (or 1/6 th of the sauce over the spaghetti.) Sprinkle 1 Tablespoon of Parmesan cheese over the sauce.

Toast bread. Stir garlic powder into the butter and spread ½ Tablespoon on each piece of toast. Place the garlic-buttered toast under the broiler just until the butter starts to bubble. Serve the spaghetti with one slice of garlic toast each. Put extra meals in freezer containers and freeze for a later day or take to work for lunch the next day.

Divide and weigh each meal to assure the meals all weigh the same, within a few tenths of an ounce.

Sugar Free Flavored Gelatin Dessert that has no PCF's can be eaten anytime you want a snack.

1/2 of any 2 Block Snack

Breakfast - 3 Blocks

French Toast

		P	C	F
1	Egg, Whole	6.0	0	5.0
1	Egg White	4.0	0	0
-	Fat Free Cooking Spray	0	0	0
2 slices	Wheat Bread, Pepperidge Farm, light	4.0	14.0	0.5
2 T	Syrup, sugar free	0	6.0	0
1 slice	Cooked Ham, 96% extra lean	5.0	0	1.0
½ t	Butter	0	0	1.8
4 oz.	Milk 2%	4.0	5.5	2.5
1½ t	Cinnamon Sugar	0	6.0	0
		23.0	31.5	10.8
		3.2	3.5	3.6

Spray a cool skillet with fat free cooking spray and heat. Stir egg and egg white, sprinkle a little cinnamon sugar on top of egg mixture and coat the first slice of bread on both sides; place in heated skillet. Sprinkle the remaining cinnamon sugar on top of the eggs and coat the second slice of bread; place in heated skillet. Lightly brown on both sides. Remove bread from skillet and heat the Canadian bacon. You can omit the cinnamon sugar and add another tablespoon of syrup. Any egg not absorbed by the bread should be fried and served as a side dish.

Lunch - 3 Blocks

Chicken Noodle Soup and Ham Sandwich

		P	C	F
½ can	Chicken Noodle	3.7	10.0	2.5
6 slices	Honey Ham, Deli-Thin 97% lean	9.9	1.9	1.5
2 slices	Wheat Bread, Pepperidge Farm, light	4.0	14.0	0.5
½ t	Butter	0	0	1.8
½ T	Miracle Whip, regular	0	1.0	3.5
1	Lettuce Leaf, Romaine	0	0	0
1	American Cheese, fat free	5.0	2.0	0
4	Pringles Fat Free Potato Chips	0.5	3.4	0
		23.1	32.3	9.8
		3.3	3.5	3.3

1/2 of any 2 Block Snack

Dinner - 4 Blocks

Chicken Dijon with Ginger Pear Sauce for 3

		P	C	F
12 oz.	Chicken Breasts, skinless, boneless	78.0	0	4.8
-	Fat Free Cooking Spray	0	0	0
2 T	Butter	0	0	22.0
-	Salt and Pepper to taste	0	0	0
15½ oz	Pears, sliced, in juice	1.9	52.5	0
½ C	Green Onions, thinly sliced	1.0	2.4	0
1 T	Molasses	0	15.0	0
1 t	Ginger Root	0	0	0
½ T	Dijon Mustard	0	0	0
½ C	Snow Peas, raw	2.0	6.0	0
2 t	Butter	0	0	7.2
1 C	Romaine Lettuce	3.0	5.0	0
1 C	Strawberries, sliced	1.0	7.0	0
30	Grapes	0	15.0	0
1 T	Mandarin Orange Salad Dressing	0	3.0	1.1
		86.9	105.9	35.1
		12.4	11.7	11.7
		4.1	3.9	3.9

Mandarin Orange Salad Dressing: Makes 4 Tablespoons.
1 t	Canola Oil
3 T	Mandarin Orange liquid, light
1 t	Red Wine Vinegar
1 t	Cider Vinegar
1 t	Sugar

    Drain pears and reserve liquid. Set aside. Season chicken with salt and pepper.
    Spray a cool skillet with fat free cooking spray; add 2 T butter and heat. Cook chicken about 9 minutes, or until chicken is no longer pink. Remove to a platter.
    Add reserved pear liquid, green onions, molasses, ginger and mustard to skillet. Bring to a boil, scraping browned bits from pan. Reduce the heat and cook for about 2 minutes. Return chicken to skillet; add pears and heat through. Place chicken on plates and spoon on the pear sauce.
    Steam Snow Peas and melt 2 t Butter over top. Serve with salad.
    Combine salad dressing ingredients, shake well and pour 1 Tablespoon over the lettuce. Mix well, divide and place in bowls. Cut the grapes in half. Divide mandarin oranges, grapes and strawberries. Place on top of the lettuce.

    Divide and weigh each meal to assure the meals all weigh the same, within a few tenths of an ounce.
    Sugar Free Jello has no PCF's and can be eaten anytime you feel like snacking.

1/2 of any 2 Block Snack

Weight and Measurements
Results Week 4

Name _____
Weight _____
Arm _____
Chest _____
Waist _____
Hips _____
Thigh _____

Name _____
Weight _____
Arm _____
Chest _____
Waist _____
Hips _____
Thigh _____

Name _____
Weight _____
Arm _____
Chest _____
Waist _____
Hips _____
Thigh _____

Name _____
Weight _____
Arm _____
Chest _____
Waist _____
Hips _____
Thigh _____

Grocery List
Week 5

Fresh Fruits and Vegetables
Garlic Cloves
Ginger Root
Onions
Green Onions
Brussels Sprouts
Snow Peas
Carrots
Cauliflower
2 Romaine Lettuce (or mixed greens)
Celery
Potatoes
2 Tangerines
Grapes
Grapefruit
2 Lemons
Broccoli
2 qt Strawberries
Frozen Peas, small pkg.

Meats
6 Chicken Legs
16 oz Bottom Round
16 oz Fillet of Sole
15 oz Orange Roughy
(Or another white fish)
9 oz Veal Cutlets
24 oz Chicken Breasts, skinless, boneless)
Breakfast Sausage,
(Low fat made with pork and turkey)

Lunch Meats
Canadian Bacon, light
Cooked Ham, 96%
Honey Ham, Deli-Thin 97%
Roast Beef, Deli-Thin 98%

Dairy
1 ½ Dozen Eggs
Butter
Milk 2%
American Cheese reduced fat, sliced
American Cheese fat free
Swiss Cheese slices, fat free
Swiss Cheese slices, regular
Orange Juice
Cool Whip, fat free
Cheddar Cheese, fat free

Canned Fruits/Vegetables
Canned Fruits/Vegetables
1 can Green Beans
2 cans Asparagus
11 oz can Corn
3 cans Mandarin Oranges, light
Vegetarian Vegetable Soup

Nuts/Seeds
Almonds, slivered

Oils
Canola Oil
Olive Oil

Spices
Parsley
Paprika
Red Pepper Flakes

Breads
English Toasting Bread
English Muffins
Shredded Wheat Cereal
2 loaves Wheat Bread, Pepperidge Farm, light

Pringles Potato Chips, fat free
White Rice
Angel Food Cake Mix
White Flour

Miscellaneous
Syrup, Sugar Free
Jam, any flavor
Sweet Pickles, small
Dill Pickles, medium
Fat Free Cooking Spray
Miracle Whip, fat free
Miracle Whip, regular
Soy Sauce
Dry Sherry
Red Wine Vinegar
Horseradish
White Wine
Beef Bouillon Cubes
Worcestershire Sauce
Cinnamon/Sugar
Sugar Free Jello
Sugar
Heinz Ketchup
Cider Vinegar
Chicken Bouillon Cubes

Planned Meals Week 5

Breakfast - 3 Blocks

Shredded Wheat		P	C	F
1	Shredded Wheat Biscuit	2.5	16.5	1.5
3 oz.	Milk 2%	3.0	4.5	1.8
2 t	Sugar	0	8.0	0
1	Egg, Whole	6.0	0	5.0
1	Egg White	4.0	0	0
-	Fat Free Cooking Spray	0	0	0
1 slice	American Cheese, fat free	5.0	2.0	0
½ t	Butter	0	0	1.8
	20.5	31.0	10.1
	2.9	3.4	3.3

Spray a cool skillet with fat free cooking spray; add the butter and heat. Whisk the egg and egg white and pour into the heated skillet. When eggs are almost done tear up the cheese and stir into the eggs. Serve with the cereal.

Lunch - 3 Blocks

Tuna Sandwich		P	C	F
2.5 oz.	Tuna, Albacore, water packed	18.7	0	1.3
2 slices	Wheat Bread, Pepperidge Farm, light	4.0	14.0	0.5
2 T	Onion, diced	0	1.4	0.2
2	Lettuce Leaves	0	0	0
1 T	Miracle Whip, regular	0	2.0	7.0
1	Sweet Pickle, small	0	4.0	0
8	Pringles Fat Free Potato Chips	1.0	6.8	0
	23.7	28.2	9.3
	3.3	3.1	3.1

(A 9-oz. can of tuna will make 3 sandwiches)
(After draining, there is 7.5 oz of tuna.)

1/2 of any 2 Block Snack

Dinner - 4 Blocks

Fillet of Sole for 3

		P	C	F
16 oz.	Fillet of Sole	63.8	0	3.8
1½ T	Flour	1.2	8.2	0
-	Fat Free Cooking Spray	0	0	0
1 T	Butter	0	0	11.0
4 T	Heinz Ketchup	0	16.0	0
1 C	Corn	6.0	40.0	2.0
1 Can	Asparagus Spears	7.0	7.0	0
1½ T	Butter	0	0	16.5

Mandarin Orange Salad:

		P	C	F
4 C	Romaine Lettuce	12.0	20.0	0
¼ C	Mandarin Oranges, light	0.5	8.0	0
10	Grapes	0	5.0	0
3 T	Mandarin Orange Salad Dressing	0	9.0	3.3
		90.7	113.2	36.6
		12.9	12.5	12.2
		4.3	4.1	4.0

Mandarin Orange Salad Dressing: Makes 4 Tablespoons.
- 1 t   Canola Oil
- 3 T   Mandarin Orange liquid, light
- 1 t   Red Wine Vinegar
- 1 t   Cider Vinegar
- 1 t   Sugar

Thaw frozen fish in milk, or if it's fresh, soak in the milk until ready to cook. Discard the left over milk. Spray a cool skillet with fat free cooking spray; add 1 Tablespoons of butter and heat. Season fish with salt and pepper and fry until fish flakes. Heat vegetables; melt 1½ Tablespoons of butter over the top.

Combine salad dressing ingredients, shake well and pour 3 Tablespoons of dressing over the lettuce, mix well, divide and place in bowls. Cut grapes in half. Divide mandarin oranges and grapes, place on top of lettuce. (You can omit the grapes and mandarin oranges and still have a balanced meal.)

Divide and weigh each meal to assure the meals all weigh the same, within a few tenths of an ounce.

Sugar Free Flavored Gelatin Dessert that has no PCF's can be eaten anytime you feel like snacking.

1/2 of any 2 Block Snack

Breakfast - 3 Blocks

Ham and Eggs with Cheese and Grapefruit

		P	C	F
1	Egg, Whole	4.0	0	5.0
1	Egg White	4.0	0	0
-	Fat Free Cooking Spray	0	0	0
1 Slice	American Cheese, fat free	5.0	2.0	0
1 slice	Cooked Ham, 96% extra lean	5.0	0	1.0
1 slice	English Toasting Bread	3.0	14.0	1.0
1 t	Butter	0	0	3.6
½	Grapefruit	1.0	10.0	0
1 t	Sugar	0	4.0	0
		22.0	30.0	10.6
		3.1	3.3	3.5

Spray a cool skillet with non-stick spray and heat. Whisk the egg and egg white and pour into the heated skillet. When the egg is almost done tear up the cheese and stir into the egg mixture until melted. Heat the ham. Toast the bread and spread with butter. Sprinkle the sugar on the grapefruit and serve.

Lunch - 3 Blocks

Roast Beef Sandwich

		P	C	F
9 slices	Roast Beef, Deli-Thin 98% lean	14.6	2.5	1.0
2 slices	Wheat Bread, Pepperidge Farm, light	4.0	14.0	0.5
2	Lettuce Leaves	0	0	0
1 T	Horseradish	0	0	0
1 T	Miracle Whip, regular	0	2.0	7.0
8	Pringles Fat Free Potato Chips	1.0	6.8	0
1	Dill Pickle, medium	0	1.0	0
		19.6	27.3	8.5
		2.8	2.9	2.8

1/2 of any 2 Block Snack

Dinner - 4 Blocks

Chicken with Orange Peel Szechwan Style for 3

		P	C	F
12 oz.	Chicken Breasts, skinless, boneless	78.0	0	4.8
-	Fat Free Cooking Spray	0	0	0
1 T	Olive Oil	0	0	14.0
3 T	Orange Peel	0.3	3.9	0.1
1 T	Soy Sauce	1.0	1.0	0
1 T	Dry Sherry	0	0	0
¼ C	Green Onions, (cut in 2" pieces)	0.5	1.2	0
¼ t	Crushed Red Pepper	0	0	0
1 t	Ginger Root, minced	0	0	0
1 T	Cornstarch	0	7.0	0
-	Salt to taste	0	0	0
½ t	Sugar	0	2.0	0
½ C	Orange Juice	0.8	13.0	0
1½ C	White Rice, cooked	6.0	57.0	0
½ C	Carrots, raw	1.0	11.5	0
½ C	Snow Peas, raw	2.0	6.0	0
1 C	Brussels Sprouts	6.0	20.0	1.0
2 T	Butter	0	0	22.0
		95.6	122.6	41.9
		13.6	13.6	13.9
		4.5	4.5	4.6

*Prepare rice as directed on the package but omit the butter.

With potato peeler, cut peel from orange and then into 1½" pieces, being careful not to cut into the white. Heat the oven to 200 degrees. Spread orange peel pieces on a cookie sheet, put in the oven, and let them dry slightly for about 30 minutes.

Cut chicken into about 1½" strips. In a medium bowl, mix chicken strips, soy sauce, green onions, sherry, red pepper and ginger. In a small bowl, mix cornstarch, salt orange juice and sugar. Cover both bowls and place in the refrigerator until you are ready to stir-fry the dinner.

Spray a cool wok with fat free cooking spray, add the oil and quickly stir-fry the slightly dried orange peel strips. Stir frequently, until peels are crisp and the edges are slightly brown. (About 2 minutes) Remove from the wok and cool on a paper towel. Add the chicken mixture to the oil in the skillet, over high heat; stir-fry the chicken until no longer pink. (About 4 minutes) Stir the orange juice mixture and add to the chicken. Stir-fry until mixture is slightly thickened. Spoon over rice; divide the orange peel and place on top of the chicken mixture and serve. Steam vegetables on separate sides of the steamer.

Divide each of the vegetable by 3 and place on plates. Divide the butter by 3 and melt over the vegetables.

Divide and weigh each meal to assure the meals all weigh the same, within a few tenths of an ounce.

Sugar Free Flavored Gelatin Dessert that has no PCF's can be eaten anytime you feel like snacking.

1/2 of any 2 Block Snack

Breakfast - 3 Blocks

French Toast with Ham   P   C   F

		P	C	F
1	Egg, Whole	6.0	0	5.0
1	Egg White	4.0	0	0
-	Fat Free Cooking Spray	0	0	0
2 slices	Wheat Bread, Pepperidge Farm, light	4.0	14.0	0.5
2 T	Syrup, sugar free	0	6.0	0
1 slice	Cooked Ham, 96% extra lean	5.0	0	1.0
½ t	Butter	0	0	1.8
4 oz.	Milk 2%	4.0	5.5	2.5
1½ t	Cinnamon Sugar	0	6.0	0
		23.0	31.5	10.8
		3.2	3.5	3.6

    Spray a cool skillet with fat free cooking spray and heat. Stir egg and egg white, sprinkle half the cinnamon sugar on top of egg mixture and coat the first slice of bread on both sides; place in heated skillet. Sprinkle the remaining cinnamon sugar on top of the eggs and coat the second slice of bread; place in heated skillet. Lightly brown on both sides. Remove bread from skillet, spread with butter and add the syrup. Heat the Ham.
    You can omit the cinnamon sugar or you can add another tablespoon of syrup. Any egg not absorbed by the bread should be fried and served as a side dish.

Lunch - 2 Blocks

Toasted Tomato Sandwich		P	C	F
2 slices	Wheat Bread, Pepperidge Farm, light	4.0	14.0	0.5
1 T	Miracle Whip, regular	0	2.0	6.0
1 T	Miracle Whip, fat free	0	2.0	0
½	Tomato, medium	0.5	3.0	0
½ C	Cottage Cheese 2%	14.0	4.0	2.0
		18.5	24.0	8.5
		2.6	2.6	2.8

1/2 of any 2 Block Snack

Dinner - 5 Blocks

Beef Stew for 4		P	C	F
16 oz.	Bottom Round, lean	107.5	0	17.2
5 T	Flour	3.7	27.5	0
-	Fat Free Cooking Spray	0	0	0
2 T	Canola Oil	0	0	28.0
¾ C	Onions, chopped	1.5	8.4	0
1	Garlic Clove, minced	0	0	0
1 t	Worcestershire Sauce	0	0	0
3 C	Water	0	0	0
-	½ t Salt, ¼ t Pepper	0	0	0
2	Beef Bouillon Cubes	0	2.0	0
10	Potatoes, New Red, 2.5" (20 oz.)	6.6	46.6	0
1 C	Carrots, diced	2.0	23.0	0
1 C	Peas, frozen	8.0	18.0	0
8 slices	Wheat Bread, Pepperidge Farm, light	18.6	58.6	2.6
1½ T	Butter	0	0	16.5
		147.9	184.1	64.3
		21.1	20.4	21.4
		5.2	5.1	5.3

    Cut beef into 1 to 1½" pieces. Coat meat with flour. Shake off excess flour and reserve. Spray a Dutch oven with fat free cooking spray, add the oil, and brown the meat all over, a few pieces at a time, removing them as they brown.

    Reduce heat to medium. To the drippings in pan, add onions and garlic. Cook 3 minutes, stirring until onions are almost tender. Stir in reserve flour. Combine Worcestershire Sauce, Beef Bouillon Cube, Water, and the Salt and Pepper. Gradually add to mixture in the pan. Cook, stirring, until slightly thickened.

    Return the meat to the pan and bring to a boil, stirring. Reduce heat to low, cover, and simmer for 2½ hours, or until the meat is tender, stirring occasionally.

    Add potatoes and carrots. Bring to a boil, reduce heat to low, cover and simmer another 20 minutes. Add the peas, cover and simmer until vegetables and meat are tender. Serve two slices of bread per person.

    Makes about 5 cups of beef stew. Serves about 1 ¼ C of beef stew with 2 slices of bread per person.

    Divide and weigh each meal to assure the meals all weigh the same, within a few tenths of an ounce.

    Sugar Free Flavored Gelatin Dessert that has no PCF's can be eaten anytime you feel like snacking.

1/2 of any 2 Block Snack

Breakfast - 3 Blocks

Eggs with Toast and Jam

		P	C	F
1	Egg, Whole	6.0	0	5.0
1	Egg White	4.0	0	0
-	Fat Free Cooking Spray	0	0	0
1 Slice	American Cheese, fat free	5.0	2.0	0
4 oz.	Milk 2%	4.0	5.5	2.5
2 oz.	Orange Juice	0.5	6.5	0
2 slice	Wheat Toast, Pepperidge Farm, light	4.0	14.0	0.5
1 t	Jam, light	0	3.0	0
½ t	Butter	0	0	1.8
		23.5	31.0	9.8
		3.3	3.4	3.2

Spray a cool skillet with fat free cooking spray and heat. Whisk the egg and egg white and pour into the skillet. When eggs are almost done tear up the cheese and stir into the scrambled eggs. Toast the bread. Spread one piece of toast with the butter and the other with jam.

Lunch - 2 Blocks

Grilled Ham and Cheese Sandwich

		P	C	F
2 slices	Wheat Bread, Pepperidge Farm, light	4.0	14.0	0.5
2 slices	American Cheese, reduced fat	8.0	4.0	6.0
½ T	Miracle Whip, fat free	0	1.0	0
1 slice	Cooked Ham, 96% extra lean	5.0	0	1.0
4	Pringles Fat Free Potato Chips	0.5	3.4	0
-	Salt and Pepper to taste	0	0	0
		17.5	22.4	7.5
		2.5	2.5	2.5

Spray a skillet with non-stick spray and grill sandwich until golden brown. Serve with chips.

1/2 of any 2 Block Snack

Dinner - 5 Blocks

Chicken Drumsticks with Angel Food Cake for 3		P	C	F
6	Chicken Legs, skinless (about 15 oz.)	87.0	0	15.0
2 T	White Flour	1.5	11.0	0
-	Fat Free Cooking Spray	0	0	0
2 T	Butter	0	0	22.0
1 can	Asparagus	7.0	7.0	0
1 C	Cauliflower, raw	2.0	5.0	0
½ C	Snow Peas, raw	2.0	6.0	0
1 T	Butter	0	0	11.0
Dessert:				
3 slices	1/12th Angel Food Cake	9.0	90.0	0
2 C	Strawberries, sliced	2.0	14.0	0
		110.5	133.0	48.0
		15.7	14.7	16.0
		5.2	4.9	5.3

Bake an Angel Food Cake mix. Divide into 12 equal pieces. (The extra pieces can be frozen, or try one of the other recipes that serve Angel Food Cake, strawberries and/or fat free Cool Whip for dessert.)

Boil chicken legs until tender, remove skin then coat with flour. Spray cool skillet with the fat free cooking spray, add 2 Tablespoon of butter, add chicken and fry until brown. (The chicken will weigh about 15 ounces after bone is removed.) (Most chicken legs will weigh about 5 ounces each with bone in.)

Steam vegetables, and melt 1 Tablespoon of butter on top.

Serve Angel food cake and strawberries for dessert.

(1 Cup of canned Peaches, light, or 2 fresh peaches, can be substituted for the strawberries and still be balanced. Or try another substitution.)

Divide and weigh each meal to assure the meals all weigh the same, within a few tenths of an ounce.

Sugar Free Flavored Gelatin Dessert that has no PCF's can be eaten anytime you feel like snacking.

1/2 of any 2 Block Snack

Breakfast - 3 Blocks

Eggs Benedict		P	C	F
1	Egg, Whole	6.0	0	5.0
1	Egg, White	4.0	0	0
-	Fat Free Cooking Spray	0	0	0
2 slices	Canadian Bacon, 97% lean	5.0	0.5	0.7
½	English Muffin	2.5	12.5	0.5
3	Potatoes, New, small (6 oz.)	1.9	13.9	0
Hollandaise Sauce:				
1	Egg Yolk	3.0	0	5.0
2 t	Lemon Juice	0	0.8	0
3 T	2% Milk	0	0	0
		22.4	27.7	11.2
		3.2	3.0	3.7

Peel potatoes, slice thinly and fry. Spray a cool skillet with fat free cooking spray and cook the egg and egg white, being careful not to break the yolk.

Hollandaise Sauce:
Place egg yolk and milk in top of double boiler. Cook over boiling water, stirring rapidly, until mixture thickens. (Water in the bottom of the double boiler should not touch the top pan.) Remove pan from water; stir rapidly for 2 minutes. Stir in 1 teaspoon of lemon juice at a time. Season with salt and white pepper to taste. Heat again over boiling water, stirring constantly, until thickened. (2 or 3 minutes.) Remove from water at once. If the Hollandaise sauce curdles immediately beat in 1 or 2 t boiling water.
Place ½ English Muffin on the plate, layers with Canadian Bacon, and then egg. Pour Hollandaise Sauce over top. Serve with fried potatoes.

Lunch - 3 Blocks

Vegetarian Vegetable Soup & Ham Sandwich		P	C	F
½ Can	Vegetarian Vegetable	3.7	20.0	1.2
2 slices	Wheat Bread, Pepperidge Farm, light	2.0	7.0	0
1½ slices	American Cheese, fat free	7.5	3.0	0
1½ slices	Cooked Ham, 96% extra lean	7.5	0	1.5
1 T	Miracle Whip, regular	0	2.0	7.0
-	Salt and Pepper to taste	0	0	0
		20.7	32.0	9.7
		2.9	3.5	3.2

1/2 of any 2 Block Snack

Dinner - 4 Blocks

Veal with Vegetables and Gravy for 3

		P	C	F
9 oz.	Veal Cutlets (3 oz. each)	67.5	0	15.6
2 T	Flour, white	1.5	11.0	0
½ T	Canola Oil	0	0	7.0
-	Non-Stick Spray	0	0	0
1 C	Carrots, sliced	2.0	23.0	0
6	Potatoes, New Red, small (12 oz.)	4.0	27.8	0
½ C	Onions, chopped	0.9	5.6	0.1
1	Celery Stalk, chopped	0	2.0	0
1 T	Butter	0	0	11.0
1 C	White Wine	0	0	0
1 C	Water	0	0	0
1 t	Parsley, dried	0	0	0
3 C	Romaine Lettuce	9.0	15.0	0
¼ C	Mandarin Oranges	0.5	8.0	0
1 C	Strawberries, sliced	1.0	7.0	0
10	Grapes	0	5.0	0
2 T	Mandarin Orange Salad Dressing	0	6.0	2.2
		86.4	110.4	35.9
		12.3	12.2	11.9
		4.1	4.0	3.9

Mandarin Orange Salad Dressing:

1 t	Canola Oil
3 T	Mandarin Orange liquid, light
1 t	Red Wine Vinegar
1 t	Cider Vinegar
1 t	Sugar

Place veal between 2 pieces of wax paper and pound lightly. Make small incisions around the edges of the cutlets to prevent them from rolling while they cook. Coat veal with flour. Shake off excess flour and reserve.

Spray skillet with fat free cooking spray; add the oil and heat. Add the onions, carrots and celery. Cook over medium heat for 3 minutes, stirring frequently. Add the veal and brown on all sides. Mix together the wine, water and reserved flour. Add to the skillet. Make sure the meat is covered with the wine mixture. Simmer over low heat for about 30 minutes or until the meat is tender. Sprinkle with parsley. Salt and pepper to taste. When ready to serve the sauce should be thick and creamy.

Combine salad dressing ingredients, shake well and pour 2 Tablespoons over the lettuce. Mix well, divide and place in bowls. Cut Grapes in half. Divide mandarin oranges, strawberries and grapes. Place on top of the lettuce. (You can omit the strawberries, grapes or mandarin oranges and still have a balanced meal.)

Divide and weigh each meal to assure the meals all weigh the same, within a few tenths of an ounce.
Sugar Free Flavored Gelatin Dessert that has no PCF's can be eaten anytime you feel like snacking.

1/2 of any 2 Block Snack

Breakfast - 3 Blocks

Sausage and Eggs with Potatoes and Jam		P	C	F
1	Egg, Whole	6.0	0	5.0
1	Egg White	4.0	0	0
-	Fat Free Cooking Spray	0	0	0
2	Potato, small red (4 oz.)	1.2	9.2	0
½ med.	Tomato, slices	0.5	3.0	0
2	Breakfast Sausage, 97% fat free	0	0	0
-	(Made with pork and turkey)	7.0	3.0	1.5
1 slice	Wheat Toast, Pepperidge Farm, light	2.0	7.0	0
3 oz.	Milk 2%	3.0	1.8	1.8
2 t	Jam, light	0	6.0	0
½ t	Butter	0	0	1.8
		23.7	30.0	10.1
		3.3	3.3	3.3

Spray a cool skillet with fat free cooking spray and heat. Peel potatoes, slice thinly and fry.
Spray another skillet and add the egg and egg white. Heat the sausage. Toast the bread and spread with butter and jam. Serve with sliced tomatoes.

Lunch - 3 Blocks

Ham & American Cheese Sandwich (Grapes)		P	C	F
8 slices	Honey Ham, Deli-Thin 97% lean	13.3	2.6	2.0
2 slices	Wheat Bread, Pepperidge Farm, light	4.0	14.0	0.5
1 T	Miracle Whip, regular	0	2.0	7.0
1	Lettuce Leaf, Romaine	0	0	0
1	American Cheese, fat free	5.0	2.0	0
5	Grapes	0	2.5	0
8	Pringles Fat Free Potato Chips	1.0	6.8	0
		23.3	29.9	9.5
		3.3	3.3	3.1

1/2 of any 2 Block Snack

Dinner - 4 Blocks

Fish and Chips for 3   P   C   F
15 oz.   Orange Roughy (or any other white fish)   60.0   0   3.7
-               Fat Free Cooking Spray   0   0   0
2 T   Butter   0   0   22.0
1½ t   Lemon Juice   0   0.5   0
-               Salt   0   0   0

-               Non-Stick Spray   0   0   0
12   Red Potatoes (or about 24 oz.)   7.7   55.7   0
-               Salt and Pepper to taste   0   0   0

6 T   Heinz Ketchup   0   24.0   0

Mandarin Orange Salad:
2 C   Romaine Lettuce   6.0   10.0   0
¼ C   Mandarin Oranges, light   0.5   8.0   0
10   Grapes   0   5.0   0
1 C   Strawberries, sliced   1.0   7.0   0
1 T   Almonds, slivered   3.0   3.0   8.0
2 T   Mandarin Orange Salad Dressing   0   6.0   2.2
                                                                    78.2   119.2   35.9
                                                                    11.1   13.2   11.9
                                                                     3.7   4.4   3.9

Mandarin Orange Salad Dressing:
1 t   Canola Oil
3 T   Mandarin Orange liquid, light
1 t   Red Wine Vinegar
1 t   Cider Vinegar
1 t   Sugar

Preheat oven to 500 degrees

Spray 2 large cookie sheets with fat free cooking spray. Wash potatoes, cut out eyes and slice to ¼" thick. Place potatoes in a bowl and toss with the salt and pepper. Divide potato slices evenly between pans. Bake about 20 minutes or until tender and lightly browned.

Thaw frozen fish in milk, or if it's fresh, soak in the milk until ready to cook. Discard the left over milk. Spray a cool skillet with non-stick spray and add 2 T butter. Heat skillet; sprinkle the fish with salt and pepper and fry fish until the fish flakes. (7 to 10 minutes.)

Divide and weigh each meal to assure the meals all weigh the same, within a few tenths of an ounce.

Sugar Free Flavored Gelatin Dessert that has no PCF's can be eaten anytime you feel like snacking.
1/2 of any 2 Block Snack

Breakfast - 2 Blocks

Poached Egg with English Toasting Bread

		P	C	F
1	Egg, Whole	6.0	0	5.0
-	Fat Free Cooking Spray	0	0	0
2 slices	Canadian Bacon, 97% lean	5.5	0	0.7
1 slice	English Toasting Bread	3.0	14.0	1.0
2 t	Jam, light	0	6.0	0
2 oz.	Milk 2%	2.0	2.7	1.2
		16.5	22.7	7.9
		2.3	2.5	2.6

Heat some water in a skillet and poach the egg. Heat the bacon. Toast the bread and spread with jam.

Lunch - 3 Blocks

Tuna Melt

		P	C	F
2 oz.	Tuna, water packed	14.9	0	1.0
1 T	Green Onions, chopped	0.1	0.3	0
2 T	Miracle Whip, fat free	0	4.0	0
2 slices	Wheat Bread, Pepperidge Farm, light	4.0	14.0	0.5
1 slices	Swiss Cheese slice, regular	4.0	1.0	5.0
1 t	Butter	0	0	3.6
1	Sweet Pickle, small	0	4.0	0
6	Pringles Fat Free Potato Chips	0.7	6.0	0
2	Strawberry, large	0	1.0	0
		23.7	30.3	10.1
		3.3	3.3	3.3

Spray a cool skillet with fat free cooking spray.

Weigh out 2 ounces of tuna; add the green onions and miracle whip. Blend well. Spread the tuna salad on the bread; spread the butter on the outside of the slices and fry in the skillet until golden brown. Serve with a sweet pickle, strawberries, and fat free chips

1/2 of any 2 Block Snack

Dinner -5 Blocks

Chicken Cordon Bleu for 3

		P	C	F
12 oz.	Chicken Breasts, skinless boneless	78.0	0	4.8
2 T	White Flour	1.4	11.0	0
1 t	Paprika	0	0	0
2½ T	Butter	0	0	27.5
-	Fat Free Cooking Spray	0	0	0
3 slices	Swiss Cheese, fat free	15.0	6.0	0
3 slices	Honey Ham Hillshire Farm 97% lean	5.0	1.0	0.7
½ C	White Wine	0	0	0
2	Chicken Bouillon Cubes	0	2.0	0
1 T	Corn Starch	0	7.0	0
1 C	Milk 2%	8.0	11.0	5.0
8	Red Potatoes, small (16 oz. peeled)	4.0	28.0	0
¼ C	Cheddar Cheese, fat free, grated	8.0	1.0	1.5
2 T	Green Onions, chopped	0	0.6	0
1 T	Butter	0	0	11.0
1 Can	Green Beans (14.5 oz.)	1.5	7.0	0
2	Tangerines	0	18.0	0
1½ C	Strawberries, diced	1.5	10.5	0
1½ C	Whipped Topping, fat free	0	48.0	0
		122.4	151.1	50.5
		7.4	16.7	16.8
		5.8	5.5	5.6

Place chicken breasts between 2 pieces of wax paper and lightly pound to flatten. Spread flattened chicken breasts, roll ham and cheese together, jellyroll style, and place in center of the chicken breasts. Fold breasts over and fasten with toothpicks. Mix flour and paprika and coat chicken breasts.

Spray skillet with fat free cooking spray; add 2½ Tablespoons of butter and heat. Add chicken and cook, turning until all sides are lightly brown. Add wine and bouillon. Reduce heat to low, cover and simmer until chicken is no longer pink. Remove chicken; pull out the toothpicks and cover to keep warm.
Mix cornstarch and milk. Add to the drippings in pan and stir until mixture thickens. Return the chicken to the pan and heat. Place chicken on the plates, divide the gravy and pour over the chicken.

While chicken is cooking, peel potatoes, dice and steam. Mash the potatoes; stir in cheddar cheese, green onions, and 1 Tablespoon of butter. Keep warm until ready to serve. Heat the green beans.
Divide and weigh each meal to assure the meals all weigh the same, within a few tenths of an ounce.

Sugar Free Flavored Gelatin Dessert that has no PCF's can be eaten anytime you feel like snacking.
1/2 of any 2 Block Snack

**Weight and Measurements
Results Week 5**

Name _____
Weight _____
Arm   _____
Chest _____
Waist _____
Hips   _____
Thigh _____

Name   _____
Weight _____
Arm   _____
Chest _____
Waist _____
Hips   _____
Thigh _____

Name   _____
Arm   _____
Chest _____
Waist _____
Hips   _____
Thigh _____

Name   _____
Weight _____
Arm   _____
Chest _____
Waist _____
Hips   _____
Thigh _____

Grocery List
Week 6

Fresh Fruits/Vegetables
6 C Strawberries
Grapes
2 Grapefruit
Onions
3 Green Peppers
Romaine Lettuce (or Mixed Greens)
1 Tomato
Cabbage
Red Potatoes
Broccoli
1 C Fresh Mushrooms
Garlic Cloves
Ginger Root
2 Peaches

Meat
12 oz Pork Loin
12 oz Orange Roughy (or any other white fish)
12 oz Veal
Turkey Breast, small
33 oz Chicken Breasts (skinless, boneless)
9 oz Tuna Albacore water pack
9 oz Beef Flank Steak

Lunch Meats
Canadian Bacon, lean
Cooked Ham 96%
Honey Ham, Deli-Thin 97%
Corned Beef, Deli-Thin

Canned Fruits/Vegetables
1 can Corn
1 can Asparagus
2 cans Green Beans
Mandarin Oranges, light
Pineapple Rings in juice, small can
Chicken Noodle Soup
Sauerkraut

Dairy
1 Doz. Eggs
Milk 2%
American Cheese, fat free
Cheddar Cheese, reduced fat
Provolone Cheese
Swiss Cheese slices, fat free
Orange Juice
Cool Whip, fat free

Breads/Starches
White Flour
English Toasting Bread
1 Wheat Bread, Pepperidge Farm, light
Special K Cereal
Pumpernickel Bread
White Rice
Fat Free Potato Chips
Manny's Tortillas, flour (6") or one with 1 P, 11 C, 1 F
Smart Start Cereal
Angel Food Cake
Cornstarch

Oils
Canola Oil
Olive Oil

Spices
Nutmeg
Paprika
Parsley
Ginger, Powder
Sugar
Chicken Bouillon Cube

Miscellaneous
White Wine
Red Wine
Thousand Island Dressing, fat free
Cider Vinegar
Soy Sauce
Horseradish
Pace Salsa
Heinz Ketchup
Open Pit Original B.B.Q. Sauce
Dill Pickle
Sweet Pickle
Jam, any flavor
Sugar Free Jello
Mustard
Red Wine Vinegar
Spinach, frozen
Miracle Whip, regular
Miracle Whip, fat free

Planned Meals Week 6

Breakfast - 3 Blocks

Eggs with Ham and Cheese

		P	C	F
1	Egg, Whole	6.0	0	5.0
-	Fat Free Cooking Spray	0	0	0
1 Slice	American Cheese, fat free	5.0	2.0	0
1 slice	English Toasting Bread	3.0	14.0	1.0
1 slice	Cooked Ham, 96% extra lean	5.0	0	1.0
2 oz	Milk 2%	2.0	2.7	1.2
3 oz.	Orange Juice	0.7	9.7	0
½ t	Butter	0	0	1.8
		21.7	28.4	10.0
		3.1	3.1	3.3

Spray a cool skillet with fat free cooking spray. Whisk the egg and scramble in the skillet. When the egg is almost done tear up the cheese and stir into the egg. Heat the ham. Toast the bread and spread with the butter.

Lunch - 3 Blocks

Tuna Sandwich

		P	C	F
2.5 oz.	Tuna, Albacore, water packed	18.7	0	1.3
2 slices	Wheat Bread, Pepperidge Farm, light	4.0	14.0	0.5
2 T	Onion, diced	0	1.4	0.2
2	Lettuce Leaves	0	0	0
1 T	Miracle Whip, regular	0	2.0	7.0
1	Sweet Pickle, small	0	4.0	0
8	Pringles Fat Free Potato Chips	1.0	6.8	0
		23.7	28.2	9.3
		3.3	3.1	3.1

Weigh out 2.5 ounces of tuna; add the diced onions and miracle whip. Blend well. Spread the tuna salad on the bread and add the lettuce. Serve with a sweet pickle and chips.

(9-oz. can of tuna makes 3 sandwiches)
(After draining, there is 7.5 oz of tuna.)

1/2 of any 2 Block Snack

Dinner - 4 Blocks

Chicken with Peach Sauté for 3

		P	C	F
12 oz.	Chicken Breasts, skinless, boneless	78.0	0	4.8
-	Fat Free Cooking Spray	0	0	0
2½ T	Canola Oil	0	0	35.0
2 oz.	Orange Juice	0.4	6.5	0
2 T	Sugar	0	24.0	0
2 t	Cornstarch	0	4.6	0
½ t	Ginger	0	0	0
¼ t	Paprika	0	0	0
-	Pepper to taste	0	0	0
¼ C	Green Pepper, wedges	0.2	2.8	0
¼ C	Onions, wedged	0.5	2.8	0
1 C	Peaches, sliced thin	1.2	16.2	0
1½ C	White Rice, cooked	6.0	57.0	0
1 Can	Green Beans	3.5	10.5	0
		90.1	124.4	39.8
		12.8	13.8	13.2
		4.2	4.6	4.4

Prepare rice as directed on package but omit the butter.

In a small bowl, combine orange juice, sugar, cornstarch, ginger, paprika and pepper to taste. Blend well and set aside. Heat oil in wok on medium high heat. Add chicken; cook 4 to 6 minutes or until lightly brown, stirring continuously. Add peppers and onions. Cook and stir 4 to 5 minutes more or until chicken is no longer pink and the vegetables are crisp-tender.

Stir the orange juice mixture and pour over the chicken. Add the peaches and cook another 2 or 3 minutes, until the sauce is thick and bubbly. Serve over rice. Heat green beans.

Divide and weigh each meal to assure the meals all weigh the same, within a few tenths of an ounce.

Sugar Free Flavored Gelatin Dessert that has no PCF's can be eaten anytime you feel like snacking.

1/2 of any 2 Block Snack

Breakfast - 2 Blocks

Poached Egg with English Toasting Bread

		P	C	F
1	Egg, Whole	6.0	0	5.0
-	Fat Free Cooking Spray	0	0	0
2 slices	Canadian Bacon, 97% lean	5.5	0	0.7
1 slice	English Toasting Bread	3.0	14.0	1.0
2 t	Jam, light	0	6.0	0
2 oz.	Milk 2%	2.0	2.7	1.2
		16.5	22.7	7.9
		2.3	2.5	2.6

Heat water and poach the egg. Heat the bacon and serve with toast and jam.

Lunch - 4 Blocks

Reuben Sandwich

		P	C	F
8 slices	Corned Beef, Deli-Thin, lean	15.2	1.8	2.6
2 slices	Pumpernickel Bread	6.0	23.6	2.0
1 slice	Swiss Cheese, fat free	5.0	3.0	0
¼ C	Sauerkraut	0	2.0	0
2 T	Thousand Island Dressing, fat free	0	6.0	0
1 T	Miracle Whip, fat free	0	2.0	0
2 t	Butter	0	0	7.3
1	Dill Pickle, medium	0	1.0	0
		26.2	39.4	11.9
		3.7	4.3	3.9

Spray a cool skillet with fat free cooking spray. Make the sandwich; blend the dressing and miracle whip, spread on the bread. Spread 1-teaspoon of butter on the outside of both slices of bread and grill until golden brown. Serve with a dill pickle.

1/2 of any 2 Block Snack

Dinner - 4 Blocks

		P	C	F
Boneless BBQ Pork" Ribs" for 3				
12 oz.	Pork Loin, boneless	68.0	0	20.0
¾ C	Barbecue Sauce	0	66.0	0
1 can	Green Beans	3.5	10.5	0
Cole Slaw:				
2 C	Cabbage, shredded	2.0	6.6	0
4 T	Miracle Whip, regular	0	4.0	14.0
1 T	Milk 2%	0.5	0.7	0.3
1 t	Cider Vinegar	0	0	0
2 t	Sugar	0	8.0	0
		74.0	95.8	34.3
		10.5	10.6	11.4
		3.5	3.5	3.8

Trim all visible fat from the boneless pork loin then slice it in half, horizontally. Cut each half crosswise into strips.

Toss ribs in barbecue sauce to coat and let stand covered until ready to grill.

Heat grill. Add ribs to grill and cook until they are lightly browned on the outside and just lose their pink in the center. (About 5 minutes, turning once.)

Heat green beans. Make the Cole Slaw and divide in 3.

Divide and weigh each meal to assure the meals all weigh the same, within a few tenths of an ounce.

Sugar Free Flavored Gelatin Dessert that has no PCF's can be eaten anytime you feel like snacking.

1/2 of any 2 Block Snack

Breakfast - 3 Blocks

Smart Start Cereal		P	C	F
2/3 C	Smart Start	2.0	27.3	0.3
3 oz.	Milk 2%	3.0	4.5	1.8
-	Fat Free Cooking Spray	0	0	0
1	Egg, Whole	6.0	0	5.0
1	Egg, White	4.0	0	0
1 t	Butter	0	0	3.6
½ slice	American Cheese, fat free	2.7	1.0	0
½ med.	Tomato, slices	0.5	3.0	0
2 slices	Canadian bacon	5.5	0	0.7
	23.2	35.8	11.4
	3.3	3.9	3.8

Spray a cool skillet with fat free cooking spray. Whisk the egg and egg white and pour into the skillet. When the eggs are almost done tear up the cheese and stir into the scrambled eggs. Heat the bacon. Slice the tomato and serve.

Lunch - 3 Blocks

Hot Ham & Swiss		P	C	F
2 slices	Wheat Bread, Pepperidge Farm, light	4.0	14.0	0.5
2 t	Butter	0	0	7.3
6 slices	Honey Ham, Deli-Thin 97% lean	10.0	2.0	1.5
1 slice	Swiss Cheese, fat free	8.0	1.0	0
1 slice	Onion, sliced thin	0	0	0
1 t	Horseradish	0	0	0
2 t	Mustard	0	0	0
1	Dill Pickle, medium	0	1.0	0
8	Pringles Fat Free Potato Chips	1.0	6.8	0
	23.0	24.8	9.8
	3.2	2.7	3.2

Make the sandwich, spread 1-teaspoon of butter on the outside of each slice and grill until golden brown. Serve with a dill pickle and fat free chips.

1/2 of any 2 Block Snack

Dinner - 4 Blocks

Hawaiian Chicken for 3

		P	C	F
12 oz.	Chicken Breasts (4 oz. each)	78.0	0	4.8
-	Fat Free Cooking Spray	0	0	0
2½ T	Olive Oil	0	0	34.0
3 T	Sugar	0	36.0	0
1 T	Cider Vinegar	0	0	0
1 T	Cornstarch	0	7.0	0
1 t	Soy Sauce	0.5	0.5	0
¼ t	Ginger Root	0	0	0
1	Chicken Bouillon Cube	0	1.0	0
3	Green Pepper Rings, ¼" thick	0.2	2.8	0
3	Pineapple Rings, in juice	0	21.0	0
¼ C	White Rice, raw (1 Cup cooked)	4.0	38.0	0
1 can	Green Beans	3.5	10.5	0
		86.2	116.8	38.8
		12.3	12.9	12.9
		4.1	4.3	4.3

Heat oven to 350 degrees

Prepare rice as directed on package but omit the butter.

Chicken:
Spray a cool skillet with fat free cooking spray. Add the olive oil and heat. Add the chicken to the hot skillet and brown on both sides. Transfer the chicken to an 8" x 8" x 2" baking dish and set aside.

Sauce:
Drain the pineapple, reserving the juice. Transfer the juice to a 1 C measuring cup. Add enough water to make 1 Cup of liquid. In a medium saucepan, using a wire whisk, stir together the juice mixture, sugar, vinegar, cornstarch, soy sauce, ginger and bouillon cube. Bring to a boil over medium heat. Reduce the heat and gently boil for about 4 minutes, stirring often, until it thickens.

Pour half the sauce over the chicken. Arrange the pineapple slices and pepper rings on top. Pour on the rest of the sauce mixture. Bake for 30 to 40 minutes or until the chicken is tender and no linger pink. Serve over rice with green beans.

Heat the green beans and serve.

Divide and weigh each meal to assure the meals all weigh the same, within a few tenths of an ounce.

Sugar Free Flavored Gelatin Dessert that has no PCF's can be eaten anytime you feel like snacking.

1/2 of any 2 Block Snack

Breakfast - 2 Blocks

Eggs and Grapefruit

		P	C	F
1	Egg, Whole	6.0	0	5.0
1	Egg, White	4.0	0	0
-	Fat Free Cooking Spray	0	0	0
1 slice	American Cheese, fat free	5.0	2.0	0
1 slice	Wheat Toast, Pepperidge Farm, light	2.0	7.0	0
½ t	Butter	0	0	1.8
½	Grapefruit	1.0	10.0	0
½ t	Sugar	0	2.0	0
		18.0	21.0	6.8
		2.5	2.3	2.2

Spray a cool skillet with fat free cooking spray. Whisk the egg and egg white and add to the heated skillet. Stir eggs occasionally and when almost done tear the American cheese in pieces and stir into the scrambled eggs. Toast the bread and spread on the butter. Prepare the grapefruit and sprinkle on the sugar.

Lunch - 3 Blocks

Ham Sandwich 1½ Sandwiches & Grapes

		P	C	F
9 slices	Honey Ham, Deli-Thin 97% lean	14.8	2.8	2.2
3 slices	Wheat Bread, Pepperidge Farm, light	6.0	22.0	1.0
1 t	Butter	0	0	3.6
1 T	Miracle Whip, regular	0	2.0	6.0
1	Lettuce Leaf, Romaine	0	0	0
1½	American Cheese, fat free	7.5	3.0	0
10	Grapes	0	5.0	0
4	Pringles Fat Free Potato Chips	0.5	3.4	0
		28.8	38.2	12.8
		4.1	4.2	4.2

1/2 of any 2 Block Snack

Dinner - 4 Blocks

Oriental Stir-Fry Shrimp for 3

		P	C	F
12 oz.	Shrimp, shelled	72.0	0	4.8
-	Fat Free Cooking Spray	0	0	0
2 T	Olive Oil	0	0	28.0
¼ C	Sherry, cooking	0	2.0	0
2 T	Soy Sauce	2.0	2.0	0
4 t	Corn Starch	0	9.2	0
½ t	Ginger, ground	0	0	0
½ C	Green Onions	1.0	2.5	0
¼ t	Garlic Powder	0	0	0
1 C	Broccoli	3.0	6.0	0.5
1 C	Cauliflower	2.0	5.0	0
¾ C	Snow Peas	3.0	9.0	0
½ C	Green Pepper	0.4	5.6	0
1½ C	White Rice, cooked	6.0	57.0	0
2 t	Sunflower Seeds	2.0	2.0	5.3
		91.4	100.3	38.6
		13.0	11.1	12.8
		4.3	3.7	4.2

Prepare rice as directed on package but omit the butter.

Stir together, sherry, soy sauce, cornstarch, ground ginger, salt, oregano, pepper and garlic. Add shrimp and coat well and set aside.

When ready to serve, cook rice according to directions on the box, but omit the butter. Spray a cool skillet with no-stick spray; add the oil and heat. Add the shrimp and stir-fry for about 3 minutes, or until shrimp are pink.

Remove the shrimp and add the vegetables. Stir-fry until the vegetables are crisp-tender. Return the shrimp to the skillet and heat just until hot. Divide the shrimp and rice by 3. Put shrimp mixture over rice and sprinkle with sunflower seeds.

Divide and weigh each meal to assure the meals all weigh the same, within a few tenths of an ounce.

Sugar Free Flavored Gelatin Dessert that has no PCF's can be eaten anytime you feel like snacking.

1/2 of any 2 Block Snack

Breakfast - 3 Blocks

Breakfast Tortilla

		P	C	F
1	Manny's Tortilla, flour (6")	1.0	12.0	1.0
1	Egg, Whole	6.0	0	5.0
2	Egg Whites	8.0	0	0
-	Fat Free Cooking Spray	0	0	0
2 T	Cheddar Cheese, low-fat	3.0	1.0	2.0
2 T	Pace Salsa	0	3.0	0
4 oz.	Milk 2%	4.0	5.5	2.5
3 oz.	Orange Juice	0.8	9.8	0
		22.8	31.3	10.5
		3.2	3.4	3.5

Spray a cool skillet with fat free cooking spray. Whisk the egg and egg white and fry. Heat the tortilla in a heated skillet, add the scrambled eggs and salsa to the center of the tortilla, fold and eat.

Lunch - 2 Blocks

Grilled Ham and Cheese Sandwich

		P	C	F
2 slices	Wheat Bread, Pepperidge Farm, light	4.0	14.0	0.5
2 slices	American Cheese, reduced fat	8.0	4.0	6.0
½ T	Miracle Whip, fat free	0	1.0	0
1 slice	Cooked Ham, 96% extra lean	5.0	0	1.0
-	Salt and Pepper to taste	0	0	0
4	Pringles Fat Free Potato Chips	0.5	3.4	0
		17.5	22.4	7.5
		2.5	2.5	2.5

Spray a cool skillet with fat free cooking spray. Construct the sandwich and grill until golden brown. Serve with 4 fat free potato chips.

1/2 of any 2 Block Snack

Dinner -4 Blocks

Bottom Round Roast and Vegetables for 3

		P	C	F
12 oz	Bottom Round	79.9	0	24.8
-	Fat Free Cooking Spray	0	0	0
1 T	Butter	0	0	11.0
½ t	Dried Thyme Leaves	0	0	0
½ t	Pepper	0	0	0
1	Bay Leaf	0	0	0
1 C	Carrots, sliced	2.0	23.0	0
6	Potatoes, New Red, small (12 oz.)	4.0	27.8	0
½ C	Onions, chopped	0.9	5.6	0.1
4	Pearl Onions	0.5	6.0	0
½ C	Red Wine	0	0	0
1	Dry Onion Soup Mix	0	16.0	0
2 T	Flour	1.4	11.0	0
¼ C	Mandarin Oranges, light	0.5	8.0	0
10	Grapes	0	5.0	0
1 C	Strawberries, sliced	1.0	7.0	0
2 T	Mandarin Orange Salad Dressing	0	6.0	2.2
		86.2	115.4	38.1
		12.3	12.8	12.7
		4.1	4.2	4.2

Mandarin Orange Salad Dressing: Makes 4 Tablespoons.
1 t	Canola Oil
3 T	Mandarin Orange liquid, light
1 t	Red Wine Vinegar
1 t	Cider Vinegar
1 t	Sugar

Pot Roast:

Preheat oven to 350-degrees. Wipe beef with damp paper towel. Place a piece of heavy foil in a shallow roasting pan. Center roast on foil; rub with thyme, pepper and bay leaf. Surround with potatoes and carrots. Pour the wine over the roast and sprinkle roast and vegetables with the soup mix. Seal foil at the top and sides. Roast in oven for about 1½ hours, or until fork-tender.

Remove roast from oven and transfer to a warm platter. Arrange vegetables around the roast. Strain the pan drippings, pressing any vegetable bits through a sieve into a 2-cup measure. Add wine to make 1¾ C liquid and put mixture into a saucepan. Mix flour with 2T of water until smooth. Stir into drippings in saucepan; bring to a boil, stirring with a wooden spoon. Reduce heat and simmer 3 minutes. Serve gravy over meat and vegetables.

Divide and weigh each meal to assure the meals all weigh the same, within a few tenths of an ounce. Sugar Free Flavored Gelatin Dessert that has no PCF's can be eaten anytime you feel like snacking.

1/2 of any 2 Block Snack

Breakfast - 3 Blocks

Special K Cereal

		P	C	F
1 C	Special K	6.0	21.0	0
3 oz.	Milk 2%	3.0	4.5	1.8
1 t	Sugar	0	4.0	0
1	Egg, Whole	6.0	0	5.0
-	Fat Free Cooking Spray	0	0	0
½ t	Butter	0	0	1.8
½ slice	American Cheese, fat free	2.5	1.0	0
2 slices	Canadian Bacon 97% lean	5.0	0	0.7
		22.5	30.5	9.3
		3.2	3.3	3.1

Spray a cool skillet with fat free cooking spray, add the butter and fry the egg with the cheese on the side. Heat the bacon and serve with the cereal.

Lunch - 3 Blocks

Chicken Noodle Soup & Ham Sandwich

		P	C	F
½ can	Chicken Noodle	3.7	10.0	2.5
6 slices	Honey Ham, Deli-Thin 97% lean	9.9	1.9	1.5
2 slices	Wheat Bread, Pepperidge Farm, light	4.0	14.0	0.5
½ t	Butter	0	0	1.8
½ T	Miracle Whip, regular	0	1.0	3.5
1	Lettuce Leaf, Romaine	0	0	0
1	American Cheese, fat free	5.0	2.0	0
4	Pringles Fat Free Potato Chips	0.5	3.4	0
		23.1	32.3	9.8
		3.3	3.5	3.2

1/2 of any 2 Block Snack

Dinner - 4 Blocks

Manhattan Chicken for 3 P C F

9 oz.	Chicken Breasts, skinless, boneless	58.5	0	3.6
1 slice	Wheat Bread, Pepperidge Farm, light	2.0	7.0	0
-	Fat Free Cooking Spray	0	0	0
1 T	Canola Oil	0	0	14.0
1 T	Butter	0	0	11.0
1	Egg White	4.0	0	0
1 C	Mushrooms, fresh, sliced	2.0	4.0	0
1	Garlic Clove	0	0	0
10 oz.	Frozen Spinach	6.9	9.3	0.5
½ t	Nutmeg	0	0	0
¼ C	White Wine	0	0	0
1 oz.	Provolone Cheese	7.0	1.0	5.0
1½ C	White Rice, cooked	6.0	57.0	0
1 can	Green Beans	3.0	6.0	0
1 C	Romaine Lettuce	3.0	5.0	0
1 C	Strawberries, sliced	1.0	7.0	0
10	Grapes	0	5.0	0
1 T	Mandarin Orange Salad Dressing	0	3.0	1.1
		93.4	104.3	35.2
		13.3	11.5	11.7
		4.4	3.8	3.9

Mandarin Orange Salad Dressing: Makes 4 Tablespoons.

1 t	Canola Oil
3 T	Mandarin Orange liquid, light
1 t	Red Wine Vinegar
1 t	Cider Vinegar
1 t	Sugar

Prepare rice as directed on package but omit the butter.

Combine salad dressing ingredients, shake well and pour 1 Tablespoon over the lettuce. Mix well, divide and place in bowls. Cut grapes in half. Divide strawberries and grapes and place on top of lettuce.

Spray a cool skillet with fat free cooking spray. Add oil and butter. Heat. Toast the bread and crumble as fine as you can. Coat the chicken with egg and then the breadcrumbs. Place chicken in skillet and brown all over. Add next 5 ingredients. Cook until chicken is no longer pink and the juices run clear. Place cheese on top of chicken breasts, cover and heat until cheese melts. Serve over rice. Heat green beans.

Divide and weigh each meal to assure the meals all weigh the same, within a few tenths of an ounce.

Sugar Free Flavored Gelatin Dessert that has no PCF's can be eaten anytime you feel like snacking.

1/2 of any 2 Block Snack

Breakfast - 3 Blocks

Ham and Eggs with Grapefruit		P	C	F
1	Egg, Whole	4.0	0	5.0
1	Egg White	4.0	0	0
-	Fat Free Cooking Spray	0	0	0
1 slice	American Cheese, fat free	5.0	2.0	0
1 slice	Cooked Ham, 96% extra lean	5.0	0	1.0
1 slice	English Toasting Bread	3.0	14.0	1.0
1 t	Butter	0	0	3.6
½	Grapefruit	1.0	10.0	0
1 t	Sugar	0	4.0	0
		22.0	30.0	10.6
		3.1	3.3	3.5

Spray a cool skillet with fat free cooking spray. Whisk the egg and egg white and add to the heated skillet. Stir eggs occasionally and when almost done tear the American cheese in pieces and stir into the scrambled eggs.

Lunch - 3 Blocks

B.L.T. with Cheese		P	C	F
2 slices	Wheat Bread, Pepperidge Farm, light	4.0	14.0	0.5
2 slice	American Cheese, fat free	10.0	4.0	0
1 leaf	Romaine Lettuce	0	0	0
½	Tomato, medium	0.5	2.0	0
3 slices	Bacon, lean	5.8	0	9.4
2 T	Miracle Whip, fat free	0	4.0	0
1	Sweet Pickle, small	0	4.0	0
		20.3	28.0	9.9
		2.9	3.1	3.3

1/2 of any 2 Block Snack

Dinner - 4 Blocks

Steak and Fries for 3		P	C	F
9 oz.	Beef Flank Steak	69.3	0	25.6
1 t	Cracked Black Pepper	0	0	0
1	Garlic Clove, small	0	0	0
½ t	Parsley	0	0	0
½ T	Canola Oil	0	0	7.0
-	Non-Stick Spray	0	0	0
12	Red Potatoes (or about 24 oz.)	7.7	55.7	0
-	Salt	0	0	0
-	Pepper	0	0	0

Mandarin Orange Salad:

1 C	Romaine Lettuce	3.0	5.0	0
½ C	Mandarin Oranges, light	1.0	16.0	0
15	Grapes	0	7.5	0
2 C	Strawberries, sliced	2.0	14.0	0
1 T	Sugar	0	9.0	0
2 T	Mandarin Orange Salad Dressing	0	6.0	2.2
		83.0	113.2	34.8
		11.8	12.5	11.6
		3.9	4.1	3.8

Mandarin Orange Salad Dressing:

1 t	Canola Oil
3 T	Mandarin Orange liquid, light
1 t	Red Wine Vinegar
1 t	Cider Vinegar
1 t	Sugar

Fries:

Preheat oven to 500 degrees. Spray 2 large cookie sheets with fat free cooking spray. Wash potatoes, cut out eyes and slice to ¼" thick. Place potatoes in a bowl and toss with the salt and pepper. Divide potato slices evenly between pans. Bake about 20 minutes or until tender and lightly browned.

Place flank steak on a plate and rub with pepper and garlic. Heat Grill on medium high. Grill steak about 14 minutes for medium-rare or until desired doneness, turning once.

Remove steak to cutting board and thinly slice steak diagonally across the grain.

Divide and weigh each meal to assure the meals all weigh the same, within a few tenths of an ounce. (You can omit the grapes and still have a balanced meal.)

Sugar Free Flavored Gelatin Dessert that has no PCF's can be eaten anytime you feel like snacking.

1/2 of any 2 Block Snack

**Weight and Measurements
Results Week 6**

Name   _____
Weight   _____
Arm   _____
Chest   _____
Waist   _____
Hips   _____
Thigh   _____

Name   _____
Weight   _____
Arm   _____
Chest   _____
Waist   _____
Hips   _____
Thigh   _____

Name   _____
Weight   _____
Arm   _____
Chest   _____
Waist   _____
Hips   _____
Thigh   _____

Name   _____
Weight   _____
Arm   _____
Chest   _____
Waist   _____
Hips   _____
Thigh   _____

Weight and Measurements
Results Week 7

Name _____
Weight _____
Arm   _____
Chest _____
Waist _____
Hips   _____
Thigh _____

Name _____
Weight _____
Arm   _____
Chest _____
Waist _____
Hips   _____
Thigh _____

Name _____
Weight _____
Arm   _____
Chest _____
Waist _____
Hips   _____
Thigh _____

Name _____
Weight _____
Arm   _____
Chest _____
Waist _____
Hips   _____
Thigh _____

Weight and Measurements
Results Week 8

Name _____
Weight _____
Arm _____
Chest _____
Waist _____
Hips _____
Thigh _____

Name _____
Weight _____
Arm _____
Chest _____
Waist _____
Hips _____
Thigh _____

Name _____
Weight _____
Arm _____
Chest _____
Waist _____
Hips _____
Thigh _____

Name _____
Weight _____
Arm _____
Chest _____
Waist _____
Hips _____
Thigh _____

Weight and Measurements
Results Week 9

Name   _____
Weight   _____
Arm   _____
Chest   _____
Waist   _____
Hips   _____
Thigh   _____

Name   _____
Weight   _____
Arm   _____
Chest   _____
Waist   _____
Hips   _____
Thigh   _____

Name   _____
Weight   _____
Arm   _____
Chest   _____
Waist   _____
Hips   _____
Thigh   _____

Name   _____
Weight   _____
Arm   _____
Chest   _____
Waist   _____
Hips   _____
Thigh   _____

**Weight and Measurements
Results Week 10**

Name _____
Weight _____
Arm   _____
Chest _____
Waist _____
Hips _____
Thigh _____

Name _____
Weight _____
Arm   _____
Chest _____
Waist _____
Hips _____
Thigh _____

Name _____
Weight _____
Arm   _____
Chest _____
Waist _____
Hips _____
Thigh _____

Name _____
Weight _____
Arm   _____
Chest _____
Waist _____
Hips _____
Thigh _____

**Weight and Measurements
Results Week 11**

Name _____
Weight _____
Arm _____
Chest _____
Waist _____
Hips _____
Thigh _____

Name _____
Weight _____
Arm _____
Chest _____
Waist _____
Hips _____
Thigh _____

Name _____
Weight _____
Arm _____
Chest _____
Waist _____
Hips _____
Thigh _____

Name _____
Weight _____
Arm _____
Chest _____
Waist _____
Hips _____
Thigh _____

Weight and Measurements
Results Week 12

Name _____
Weight _____
Arm   _____
Chest _____
Waist _____
Hips   _____
Thigh _____

Name   _____
Weight _____
Arm   _____
Chest _____
Waist _____
Hips   _____
Thigh _____

Name   _____
Weight _____
Arm   _____
Chest _____
Waist _____
Hips   _____
Thigh _____

Name   _____
Weight _____
Arm   _____
Chest _____
Waist _____
Hips   _____
Thigh _____

Alternative Meals

Breakfast Choices

Breakfast - 2 Blocks

Cottage Cheese with Mandarin Oranges

		P	C	F
½ C	Cottage Cheese 2%	14.0	4.0	2.0
½ C	Mandarin Oranges, light	1.0	16.0	0
½ T	Almonds, slivered	2.0	2.0	4.0
		17.0	22.0	6.0
		2.4	2.4	2.0

Cottage Cheese with Fresh Peaches

		P	C	F
½ C	Cottage Cheese 2%	14.0	4.0	2.0
1 C	Peach, fresh, sliced	1.2	16.2	0
½ T	Almonds, slivered	1.5	1.5	4.0
		16.7	21.7	6.0
		2.3	2.4	2.0

Cottage Cheese with Canned Peaches

		P	C	F
½ C	Cottage Cheese 2%	14.0	4.0	2.0
½ C	Peach slices, canned, in juice	0	14.0	0
½ T	Almonds, slivered	1.5	1.5	4.0
		15.5	19.5	6.0
		2.2	2.2	2.0

Cottage Cheese with Crushed Pineapple

		P	C	F
½ C	Cottage Cheese 2%	14.0	4.0	2.0
½ C	Pineapple, crush, light	0.5	16.0	0.5
½ T	Almonds, slivered	2.0	2.0	4.0
		16.5	22.0	6.5
		2.3	2.4	2.1

Cottage Cheese with Fruit Cocktail

		P	C	F
½ C	Cottage Cheese 2%	14.0	4.0	2.0
½ C	Fruit Cocktail, light	0	14.0	0
½ T	Almonds, slivered	1.5	1.5	4.0
		15.5	19.5	6.0
		2.2	2.2	2.0

Breakfast - 2 Blocks

Cottage Cheese with Strawberries   P   C   F

		P	C	F
½ C	Cottage Cheese 2%	14.0	4.0	2.0
2 C	Strawberries	2.0	14.0	0
½ T	Almonds, slivered	1.5	1.5	4.0
		17.5	19.5	6.0
		2.5	2.2	2.0

Cottage Cheese with Blackberries

		P	C	F
½ C	Cottage Cheese 2%	14.0	4.0	2.0
1 C	Blackberries	1.0	11.2	0
½ T	Almonds, slivered	1.5	1.5	4.0
		16.5	16.7	6.0
		2.3	1.9	2.0

Cottage Cheese and Raspberries

		P	C	F
½ C	Cottage Cheese 2%	14.0	4.0	2.0
1 C	Raspberries	1.0	14.0	0
½ T	Almonds, slivered	2.0	2.0	4.0
		17.0	20.0	6.0
		2.4	2.2	2.0

Poached Egg with English Toasting Bread

		P	C	F
1	Egg, Whole	6.0	0	5.0
-	Fat Free Cooking Spray	0	0	0
2 slices	Canadian Bacon, lean	5.5	0	0.7
1 slices	English Toasting Bread	3.0	14.0	1.0
2 t	Jam, light	0	6.0	0
2 oz.	Milk 2%	2.0	2.7	1.2
		16.5	22.7	7.9
		2.3	2.5	2.6

Breakfast - 2 Blocks

Nutritionally Balanced Bar   P   C   F

| 1 | Nutritionally Balanced Bar | 2.0 | 2.0 | 2.0 |

Poached Egg with Cantaloupe   P   C   F

		P	C	F
1	Egg, Poached	6.0	0	5.0
-	Fat Free Cooking Spray	0	0	0
2 slices	Canadian Bacon, lean	5.5	0	0.7
1 slice	Wheat Bread, Pepperidge Farm, light	2.0	7.0	0
½ t	Butter	0	0	1.8
1½ C	*Cantaloupe, cubed	2.1	20.1	0.8
		15.6	27.1	8.3
		2.2	3.0	2.7

(About ¼ average cantaloupe)

Shredded Wheat

		P	C	F
1	Shredded Wheat Biscuit	2.5	16.5	1.5
3 oz.	Milk 2%	3.0	4.5	1.8
½ t	Sugar	0	2.0	0
-	Fat Free Cooking Spray	0	0	0
1	Egg, Whole	6.0	0	5.0
1 slice	American Cheese, fat free	5.0	2.0	0
		15.5	25.0	8.3
		2.4	2.7	2.7

Eggs and Grapefruit

		P	C	F
1	Egg, Whole	6.0	0	5.0
1	Egg, White	4.0	0	0
-	Fat Free Cooking Spray	0	0	0
1 slice	American Cheese, fat free	5.0	2.0	0
1 slice	Wheat Bread, Pepperidge Farm, light	2.0	7.0	0
½ t	Butter	0	0	1.8
½	Grapefruit	1.0	10.0	0
½ t	Sugar	0	2.0	0
		18.0	21.0	6.8
		2.5	2.3	2.2

Breakfast - 2 Blocks

Egg and Cheese with Strawberries

		P	C	F
1	Egg, Whole	6.0	0	5.0
-	Fat Free Cooking Spray	0	0	0
1 slice	Wheat Toast, Pepperidge Farm, light	2.0	7.0	0
1 slice	American Cheese, fat free	5.0	2.0	0
1 C	Strawberries	1.0	7.0	0
½ t	Sugar	0	2.0	0
1 t	Jam	0	3.0	0
1 t	Butter	0	0	3.6
		14.0	21.0	8.6
		2.0	2.3	2.2

Egg With Cheese

		P	C	F
1	Egg, Whole	6.0	0	5.0
-	Fat Free Cooking Spray	0	0	0
1 Slice	American Cheese, fat free	5.0	2.0	0
2 oz.	Milk 2%	2.0	2.7	1.2
2 slices	Wheat Toast, Pepperidge Farm, light	4.0	14.0	0.5
1 t	Jam, light	0	3.0	0
½ t	Butter	0	0	1.8
		17.0	21.7	8.5
		2.4	2.4	2.8

Breakfast - 3 Blocks

Sausage and Egg with Orange Juice

		P	C	F
1	Egg, Whole	6.0	0	5.0
-	Fat Free Cooking Spray	0	0	0
2	Breakfast Sausage, 97% fat free	0	0	0
-	(Made with pork and turkey)	7.0	3.0	1.5
1 slice	Wheat Bread, Pepperidge Farm, light	1.0	7.0	0
3 oz.	Milk 2%	3.0	1.8	1.8
4 oz.	Orange Juice	1.0	13.0	0
½ t	Butter	0	0	1.8
		19.0	28.5	10.1
		2.7	3.1	3.3

Nutritionally Balanced Shake

		P	C	F
2 scoops	2 Block Balance Drink Mix (any flavor)	8.0	11.0	5.0
8 oz.	2% Milk	14.0	19.0	6.0
		22.0	30.0	11.0
		3.1	3.3	3.6

Breakfast - 3 Blocks

Breakfast Tortilla

		P	C	F
1	Manny's Tortilla, flour (6")	1.0	12.0	1.0
1	Egg, Whole	6.0	0	5.0
2	Egg Whites	8.0	0	0
-	Fat Free Cooking Spray	0	0	0
2 T	Cheddar Cheese, low-fat	3.0	1.0	2.0
2 T	Pace Salsa	0	3.0	0
4 oz.	Milk 2%	4.0	5.5	2.5
3 oz.	Orange Juice	0.8	9.8	0
		22.8	31.3	10.5
		3.2	3.4	3.5

Egg and Cheese With English Toasting Bread

		P	C	F
1	Egg, Whole	6.0	0	5.0
-	Fat Free Cooking Spray	0	0	0
1 Slice	American Cheese, fat free	5.0	2.0	0
1 slice	English Toasting Bread	3.0	14.0	1.0
1 slice	Cooked Ham, 96% extra lean	5.0	0	1.0
4 oz.	Orange Juice	1.0	13.0	0
½ t	Butter	0	0	1.8
		20.0	29.0	8.8
		2.8	3.2	2.9

Omelet with Ham and Cheese

		P	C	F
1	Egg, Whole	6.0	0	5.0
-	Fat Free Cooking Spray	0	0	0
½ slice	Cooked Ham, 96% extra lean	2.5	0	0.5
1 T	Green Pepper, diced	0	0.3	0
1 T	Onion, diced	0	0.3	0
1 slice	American Cheese, fat free	5.0	2.0	0
1 T	Jam, light	0	9.0	0
2 slices	Wheat Toast, Pepperidge Farm, light	4.0	14.0	0.5
½ t	Butter	0	0	1.8
4 oz.	Milk 2%	4.0	5.5	2.5
		21.5	31.1	10.3
		3.0	3.4	3.4

Eggs with Toast and Jam

		P	C	F
1	Egg, Whole	6.0	0	5.0
1	Egg White	4.0	0	0
-	Fat Free Cooking Spray	0	0	0
1 slice	American Cheese, fat free	5.0	2.0	0
4 oz.	Milk 2%	4.0	5.5	2.5
2 oz.	Orange Juice	0.5	6.5	0
2 slice	Wheat Toast, Pepperidge Farm, light	4.0	14.0	0.5
1 t	Jam, light	0	3.0	0
½ t	Butter	0	0	1.8
		23.5	31.0	9.8
		3.3	3.4	3.2

Breakfast - 3 Blocks

Eggs with Ham and Cheese   P   C   F

		P	C	F
1	Egg, Whole	6.0	0	5.0
-	Fat Free Cooking Spray	0	0	0
1 slice	American Cheese, fat free	5.0	2.0	0
1 slice	English Toasting Bread	3.0	14.0	1.0
1 slice	Cooked Ham, 96% extra lean	5.0	0	1.0
2 oz	Milk 2%	2.0	2.7	1.2
3 oz.	Orange Juice	0.7	9.7	0
½ t	Butter	0	0	1.8
		21.7	28.4	10.0
		3.1	3.1	3.3

Eggs with Cheese and Bacon

		P	C	F
1	Egg, Whole	6.0	0	5.0
1	Egg White	4.0	0	0
-	Fat Free Cooking Spray	0	0	0
1 slice	American Cheese, fat free	5.0	2.0	0
½ med.	Tomato, slices	0.5	3.0	0
2 slices	Wheat Toast, Pepperidge Farm, light	4.0	14.0	0.5
1 slice	Bacon, lean	1.9	0	1.0
4 oz.	Orange Juice	1.0	13.0	0
2 oz.	Milk 2%	2.0	2.7	1.2
1 t	Butter	0	0	3.6
		24.4	34.7	11.3
		3.4	3.8	3.7

Eggs with Ham and Salsa

		P	C	F
1	Egg, Whole	6.0	0	5.0
1	Egg White	4.0	0	0
-	Fat Free Cooking Spray	0	0	0
2 T	Pace Salsa	0	3.0	0
1½ slices	Cooked Ham, 96% extra lean	7.5	0	1.5
3 oz.	Milk 2%	3.0	4.3	1.8
3 oz.	Orange Juice	0.8	9.8	0
2 slices	Wheat Toast, Pepperidge Farm, light	4.0	14.0	0.5
1 t	Jam, light	0	3.0	0
½ t	Butter	0	0	1.8
		25.3	34.1	10.6
		3.6	3.7	3.5

Breakfast - 3 Blocks

Eggs and Sausage with Potatoes and Jam

		P	C	F
1	Egg, Whole	6.0	0	5.0
1	Egg White	4.0	0	0
-	Fat Free Cooking Spray	0	0	0
2	Potato, small red (4 oz.)	1.2	9.2	0
½ med.	Tomato, slices	0.5	3.0	0
2	Breakfast Sausage, 97% fat free	0	0	0
-	(Made with pork and turkey)	7.0	3.0	1.5
1 slice	Wheat Toast, Pepperidge Farm, light	2.0	7.0	0
3 oz.	Milk 2%	3.0	1.8	1.8
2 t	Jam, light	0	6.0	0
½ t	Butter	0	0	1.8
		23.7	30.0	10.1
		3.3	3.3	3.3

Eggs and Sausage with Potatoes and Strawberries

		P	C	F
1	Egg, Whole	6.0	0	5.0
1	Egg White	4.0	0	0
-	Fat Free Cooking Spray	0	0	0
2	Potato, small red (4 oz.)	1.2	9.2	0
1 med.	Tomato, slices	1.0	6.0	0
1	Breakfast Sausage, 97% fat free	0	0	0
-	(Made with pork and turkey)	3.5	1.5	0.7
1 slice	Wheat Toast, Pepperidge Farm, light	2.0	7.0	0
3 oz.	Milk 2%	3.0	1.8	1.8
½ C	Strawberries	0.5	3.5	0
½ t	Butter	0	0	1.8
		21.2	29.0	9.3
		3.0	3.2	3.1

Eggs Benedict

		P	C	F
1	Egg, Whole	6.0	0	5.0
1	Egg, White	4.0	0	0
-	Fat Free Cooking Spray	0	0	0
2 slices	Canadian Bacon, 97% lean	5.0	0.5	0.7
½	English Muffin	2.5	12.5	0.5
3	Potatoes, New, small (6 oz.)	1.9	13.9	0

Hollandaise Sauce:

1	Egg Yolk	3.0	0	5.0
2 t	Lemon Juice	0	0.8	0
3 T	2% Milk	0	0	0
		22.4	27.7	11.2
		3.2	3.0	3.7

Breakfast - 3 Blocks

French Toast with Ham

		P	C	F
1	Egg, Whole	6.0	0	5.0
1	Egg White	4.0	0	0
-	Fat Free Cooking Spray	0	0	0
2 slices	Wheat Bread, Pepperidge Farm, light	4.0	14.0	0.5
2 T	Syrup, sugar free	0	6.0	0
1 slice	Cooked Ham, 96% extra lean	5.0	0	1.0
½ t	Butter	0	0	1.8
4 oz.	Milk 2%	4.0	5.5	2.5
1½ t	Cinnamon Sugar	0	6.0	0
		23.0	31.5	10.8
		3.2	3.5	3.6

Eggs with Potatoes and Sausage

		P	C	F
1	Egg, Whole	6.0	0	5.0
1	Egg White	4.0	0	0
-	Fat Free Cooking Spray	0	0	0
2	Potato, small red (4 oz.) sliced	1.2	9.2	0
-	Non-Fat Spray	0	0	0
½ med.	Tomato, slices	0.5	3.0	0
1	Breakfast Sausage, 97% fat free	0	0	0
-	(Made with pork and turkey)	3.5	1.5	0.7
2 slices	Wheat Toast, Pepperidge Farm, light	4.0	14.0	0
3 oz.	Milk 2%	3.0	1.8	1.8
1 t	Jam, light	0	3.0	0
1 t	Butter	0	0	3.6
		22.2	32.5	11.1
		3.2	3.6	3.7

Omelet with Ham and Salsa

		P	C	F
1	Egg, Whole	6.0	0	5.0
1	Egg White	4.0	0	0
-	Fat Free Cooking Spray	0	0	0
1 slice	Cooked Ham, 96% extra lean	5.0	0	1.0
1 T	Green Pepper, diced	0	0.7	0
1 T	Onion, diced	0.1	0.3	0
2 T	Pace Salsa	0	3.0	0
1 slice	American Cheese, fat free	5.0	2.0	0
2 oz.	Milk 2%	2.0	2.7	1.2
2 slices	Wheat Toast, Pepperidge Farm, light	2.0	14.0	0.5
3 oz.	Orange Juice	0.7	9.7	0
1 t	Butter	0	0	3.6
		24.8	32.7	11.3
		3.5	3.6	3.7

Breakfast - 3 Blocks

Eggs with Ham and Orange Juice   P   C   F

		P	C	F
1	Egg, Whole	6.0	0	5.0
1	Egg White	4.0	0	0
-	Fat Free Cooking Spray	0	0	0
2 slice	Wheat Toast, Pepperidge Farm, light	4.0	14.0	0.5
1½ slices	Cooked Ham, 96% extra lean	7.5	0	1.5
2 T	Pace Salsa	0	3.0	0
4 oz.	Orange Juice	1.0	13.0	0
1 t	Butter	0	0	3.6
		22.5	30.0	10.6
		3.2	3.3	3.5

Wheaties Cereal

		P	C	F
1 C	Wheaties	2.7	22.0	0.5
3 oz.	Milk 2%	3.0	4.5	1.8
1 t	Sugar	0	4.0	0
1	Egg, Whole	6.0	0	5.0
½ t	Butter	0	0	1.8
½ slice	American Cheese, fat free	2.5	1.0	0
1½ slices	Cooked Ham, 96% extra lean	7.5	0	1.5
		21.7	31.5	10.6
		3.1	3.5	3.5

Special K Cereal

		P	C	F
1 C	Special K	6.0	21.0	0
3 oz.	Milk 2%	3.0	4.5	1.8
1 t	Sugar	0	4.0	0
1	Egg, Whole	6.0	0	5.0
½ t	Butter	0	0	1.8
½ slice	American Cheese, fat free	2.5	1.0	0
2 slices	Canadian Bacon 97% lean	5.0	0	0.7
		22.5	30.5	9.3
		3.2	3.3	3.1

Cinnamon Toast Crunch Cereal

		P	C	F
1 oz.	Cinnamon Toast Crunch	1.0	21.0	3.0
4 oz.	Milk 2%	4.0	5.5	2.5
1	Egg, Whole	6.0	0	5.0
2	Egg Whites	8.0	0	0
-	Fat Free Cooking Spray	0	0	0
1 slice	American Cheese, fat free	5.0	2.0	0
		24.0	28.5	10.5
		3.4	3.1	3.5

Breakfast - 3 Blocks

Shredded Wheat | | P | C | F
1 | Shredded Wheat Biscuit | 2.5 | 16.5 | 1.5
3 oz. | Milk 2% | 3.0 | 4.5 | 1.8
2 t | Sugar | 0 | 8.0 | 0
| | | |
1 | Egg, Whole | 6.0 | 0 | 5.0
1 | Egg White | 4.0 | 0 | 0
- | Fat Free Cooking Spray | 0 | 0 | 0
1 slice | American Cheese, fat free | 5.0 | 2.0 | 0
½ t | Butter | 0 | 0 | 1.8
| | 20.5 | 31.0 | 10.1
| | 2.9 | 3.4 | 3.3

Honey Bunches of Oats with Almonds Cereal | | P | C | F
1 oz. | Honey Bunches of Oats with Almonds | 2.0 | 21.0 | 3.0
3 oz. | Milk, 2% | 3.0 | 4.5 | 1.8
| | | |
1 | Egg, Whole | 6.0 | 0 | 5.0
1 | Egg White | 4.0 | 0 | 0
- | Fat Free Cooking Spray | 0 | 0 | 0
1 slice | American Cheese, fat free | 5.0 | 2.0 | 0
| | 20.0 | 27.5 | 9.8
| | 2.8 | 3.0 | 3.2

Oatmeal | | P | C | F
½ C | Oatmeal, dry | 6.0 | 25.0 | 2.0
3 oz. | Milk 2% | 3.0 | 4.5 | 1.8
1 t | Sugar | 0 | 4.0 | 0
| | | |
1 | Egg, Whole | 6.0 | 0 | 5.0
1 | Egg, White | 4.0 | 0 | 0
½ t | Butter | 0 | 0 | 1.8
1 slice | American Cheese, fat free | 5.0 | 2.0 | 0
| | 24.0 | 35.5 | 10.6
| | 3.4 | 3.9 | 3.5

Wheat Chex Cereal | | P | C | F
¾ C | Wheat Chex | 3.7 | 26.2 | 0.7
3 oz. | Milk 2% | 3.0 | 4.5 | 1.8
1 | Egg, Whole | 6.0 | 0 | 5.0
½ t | Butter | 0 | 0 | 1.8
1 slice | American Cheese, fat free | 5.5 | 2.0 | 0
2 slices | Canadian bacon, lean | 5.5 | 0 | 0.7
| | 23.2 | 32.7 | 10.0
| | 3.3 | 3.6 | 3.3

Breakfast - 3 Blocks

Smart Start Cereal   P   C   F

		P	C	F
2/3 C	Smart Start	2.0	27.3	0.3
3 oz.	Milk 2%	3.0	4.5	1.8
1	Egg, Whole	6.0	0	5.0
1	Egg, White	4.0	0	0
1 t	Butter	0	0	3.6
½ slice	American Cheese, fat free	2.7	1.0	0
½ med.	Tomato, slices	0.5	3.0	0
2 slices	Canadian bacon, lean	5.5	0	0.7
		23.2	35.8	11.4
		3.3	3.9	3.8

Frosted Flakes Cereal

		P	C	F
¾ C	Frosted Flakes	1.0	27.0	0
3 oz.	Milk, 2%	3.0	4.5	1.8
½ t	Butter	0	0	1.8
1	Egg, Whole	6.0	0	5.0
-	Fat Free Cooking Spray	0	0	0
1 slice	American Cheese, fat free	5.0	2.0	0
2 slices	Cooked Ham, 96% extra lean	10.0	0	2.0
		25.0	33.5	10.6
		3.5	3.7	3.5

Sausage and Eggs with Cantaloupe

		P	C	F
1	Egg, Whole	4.0	0	5.0
1	Egg White	4.0	0	0
-	Fat Free Cooking Spray	0	0	0
2 T	Salsa	0	3.0	0
2	Breakfast Sausage, 97% fat free	0	0	0
-	(Made with pork and turkey)	7.0	3.0	1.5
1 slice	Wheat Toast, Pepperidge Farm, light	1.0	7.0	0
½ t	Butter	0	0	1.8
1 Cup	Cantaloupe	1.4	13.4	0.4
		17.4	26.4	8.7
		2.4	2.9	2.9

Breakfast - 3 Blocks

Ham and Eggs with Grapefruit

		P	C	F
1	Egg, Whole	4.0	0	5.0
1	Egg White	4.0	0	0
-	Fat Free Cooking Spray	0	0	0
1 slice	American Cheese, fat free	5.0	2.0	0
1 slice	Cooked Ham, 96% extra lean	5.0	0	1.0
1 slice	English Toasting Bread	3.0	14.0	1.0
1 t	Butter	0	0	3.6
½	Grapefruit	1.0	10.0	0
1 t	Sugar	0	4.0	0
		22.0	30.0	10.6
		3.1	3.3	3.5

Spray a cool skillet with fat free cooking spray and fry the egg. Heat the ham. Toast the bread and spread with butter. Serve with 1/2 grapefruit.

Breakfast - 4 Blocks

Ham and Eggs with Toast and Salsa

		P	C	F
1	Egg, Whole	6.0	0	5.0
1	Egg White	4.0	0	0
-	Fat Free Cooking Spray	0	0	0
2 slices	Wheat Toast, Pepperidge Farm, light	4.0	14.0	0.5
2 T	Pace Salsa	0	3.0	0
3 oz.	Milk 2%	3.0	4.5	1.2
4 oz.	Orange Juice	1.0	13.0	0
2 t	Jam, light	0	6.0	0
1 t	Butter	0	0	3.6
2 slices	Cooked Ham, 96% extra lean	10.0	0	2.0
		28.0	40.5	12.3
		4.0	4.5	4.1

Ham and Eggs with Toast and Strawberries

		P	C	F
1	Egg, Whole	6.0	0	5.0
1	Egg White	4.0	0	0
-	Fat Free Cooking Spray	0	0	0
2 slices	Wheat Toast, Pepperidge Farm, light	4.0	14.0	0.5
3 oz.	Milk 2%	3.0	4.5	1.2
4 oz.	Orange Juice	1.0	13.0	0
½ C	Strawberries	0.5	3.5	0
2 t	Jam, light	0	6.0	0
1 t	Butter	0	0	3.6
2 slices	Cooked Ham, 96% extra lean	10.0	0	2.0
		28.5	41.0	12.3
		4.0	4.5	4.1

Breakfast - 4 Blocks

Malt-O-Meal

		P	C	F
3 T	Malt-O-Meal (dry)	4.0	26.0	0
1 T	Wheat Germ	2.0	2.0	0.5
1 t	Sugar	0	4.0	0
3 oz.	Milk 2%	3.0	4.5	1.2
1	Egg, Whole	6.0	0	5.0
1	Egg, White	4.0	0	0
-	Fat Free Cooking Spray	0	0	0
½ t	Butter	0	0	1.8
1 slice	American Cheese, reduced fat	4.0	3.0	3.0
1 slice	Cooked Ham, 96% extra lean	5.0	0	1.0
		28.0	39.5	12.5
		4.0	4.3	4.1

Eggs with Salsa

		P	C	F
2	Eggs, Whole	12.0	0	10.0
2	Egg Whites	8.0	0	0
-	Fat Free Cooking Spray	0	0	0
2 slices	Wheat Toast, Pepperidge Farm, light	4.0	14.0	0.5
2 t	Jam, light	0	6.0	0
2 T	Pace Salsa	0	3.0	0
3 oz.	Milk 2%	3.0	4.5	1.2
4 oz.	Orange Juice	0.8	13.0	0
½ t	Butter	0	0	1.8
		27.8	40.5	13.5
		3.9	4.5	4.5

Sausage and Eggs with Milk and Orange Juice

		P	C	F
2	Eggs, Whole	12.0	0	10.0
1	Egg White	4.0	0	0
-	Fat Free Cooking Spray	0	0	0
2	Breakfast Sausage, 97% fat free	0	0	0
-	(Made with pork and turkey)	7.0	3.0	1.5
2 slices	Wheat Toast, Pepperidge Farm, light	4.0	14.0	0.5
2 t	Jam, light	0	6.0	0
2 T	Pace Salsa	0	3.0	0
2 oz.	Milk 2%	2.0	3.0	0.8
4 oz.	Orange Juice	0.8	13.0	0
½ t	Butter	0	0	1.8
		29.8	42.0	14.6
		4.2	4.6	4.8

Breakfast - 4 Blocks

Eggs with Toast and Ham

		P	C	F
1	Egg, Whole	6.0	0	5.0
1	Egg White	4.0	0	0
-	Fat Free Cooking Spray	0	0	0
2 slices	Wheat Toast, Pepperidge Farm, light	4.0	14.0	0.5
3 oz.	Milk 2%	3.0	4.5	1.2
4 oz.	Orange Juice	1.0	13.0	0
2 t	Jam, light	0	6.0	0
1 t	Butter	0	0	3.6
2 slices	Cooked Ham, 96% extra lean	10.0	0	2.0
		28.0	37.5	12.3
		4.0	4.1	4.1

Omelet with Ham and Orange Juice

		P	C	F
1	Egg, Whole	6.0	0	5.0
2	Egg Whites	8.0	0	0
-	Fat Free Cooking Spray	0	0	0
1 slice	Cooked Ham, 96% extra lean	5.0	0	1.0
1 T	Green Pepper, diced	0	0.7	0
1 T	Onion, diced	0.1	0.7	0
2 T	Cheddar Cheese, fat free	4.5	0.5	0
1 T	Celery, diced	0	0	0
2 slices	Wheat Toast, Pepperidge Farm, light	4.0	14.0	0.5
3 oz.	Milk 2%	3.0	4.5	1.2
4 oz.	Orange Juice	0.8	13.0	0
1½ t	Butter	0	0	5.4
1 t	Jam, light	0	3.0	0
		31.4	36.4	13.1
		4.4	4.0	4.3

Ham and Eggs with Salsa and English Toasting Bread

		P	C	F
1	Egg, Whole	6.0	0	5.0
2	Egg Whites	8.0	0	0
-	Fat Free Cooking Spray	0	0	0
2	English Toasting Bread	6.0	30.0	2.0
2 slices	Cooked Ham, 96% extra lean	10.0	0	2.0
2 t	Jam, light	0	6.0	0
1 T	Pace Salsa	0	1.5	0
1 t	Butter	0	0	3.6
		30.0	37.5	12.6
		4.2	4.1	4.2

Breakfast - 4 Blocks

French Toast with Sausage   P   C   F

		P	C	F
1	Egg, Whole	6.0	0	5.0
2	Egg Whites	8.0	0	0
-	Fat Free Cooking Spray	0	0	0
2 slices	Wheat Bread, Pepperidge Farm, light	4.0	14.0	0.5
2 T	Syrup, sugar free	0	6.0	0
2	Breakfast Sausage, 97% fat free	0	0	0
-	(Made with pork and turkey)	7.0	3.0	1.5
1 t	Butter	0	0	3.6
4 oz.	Milk 2%	4.0	5.5	2.5
1 T	Cinnamon Sugar	0	12.0	0
		29.0	40.5	13.1
		4.1	4.5	4.3

French Toast with Ham and Orange Juice

		P	C	F
1	Egg, Whole	6.0	0	5.0
2	Egg Whites	8.0	0	0
-	Fat Free Cooking Spray	0	0	0
2 slices	Wheat Bread, Pepperidge Farm, light	4.0	14.0	0.5
3 T	Syrup, sugar free	0	9.0	0
2 slices	Cooked Ham	10.0	0	2.0
1 t	Butter	0	0	3.6
4 oz.	Milk 2%	4.0	5.5	2.5
4 oz.	Orange Juice	0.8	13.0	0
		32.8	41.5	13.6
		4.6	4.6	4.5

Egg and Ham with English Toasting Bread

		P	C	F
1	Egg, Whole	6.0	0	5.0
2	Egg, Whites	8.0	0	0
-	Fat Free Cooking Spray	0	0	0
2 slices	English Toasting Bread	6.0	28.0	2.0
1 slice	Cooked Ham, 96% extra lean	5.0	0	1.0
2 oz.	Milk 2%	2.0	2.7	1.2
2 t	Jam, light	0	6.0	0
1 t	Butter	0	0	3.6
		27.0	36.7	12.8
		3.8	4.0	4.2

Breakfast - 4 Blocks

Omelet with Ham and Pear

		P	C	F
1	Egg, Whole	6.0	0	5.0
2	Egg Whites	8.0	0	0
-	Fat Free Cooking Spray	0	0	0
1 slice	Cooked Ham, 96% extra lean	5.0	0	1.0
2 T	Green Pepper, diced	0	0.6	0
2 T	Onion, diced	0.2	0.6	0
1 slice	American Cheese, fat free	5.0	2.0	0
¼ C	Pear, canned in own juice	0.2	7.5	0
4 oz.	Milk 2%	4.0	5.5	2.5
4 oz.	Orange Juice	0.8	13.0	0
1 slice	Wheat Toast, Pepperidge Farm, light	1.0	7.0	0
1 t	Butter	0	0	3.6
		30.2	36.2	12.1
		4.3	4.0	4.0

Eggs with Potatoes and Bacon

		P	C	F
1	Egg, Whole	6.0	0	5.0
2	Egg Whites	8.0	0	0
-	Fat Free Cooking Spray	0	0	0
1½ slice	American Cheese, fat free	7.5	3.0	0
1 slice	Bacon	1.9	0	3.1
2	Potato, small red (4 oz.) sliced	1.2	9.2	0
½ med.	Tomato, slices	0.5	3.0	0
4 oz.	Orange Juice	0.8	13.0	0
1 slice	Wheat Bread, Pepperidge Farm, light	1.0	7.0	0
1 t	Butter	0	0	3.6
		26.9	35.2	11.7
		3.8	3.9	3.9

Lunch Choices

Lunch - 2 Block

Tavern Hamburgers for 3

		P	C	F
8 oz.	Ground Beef, 93% lean	42.0	0	12.0
¼ C	Onions, diced	0.4	2.8	0
3 T	Heinz Ketchup	0	12.0	0
1 T	Soy Sauce	1.0	1.0	0
½ T	Cider Vinegar	0	0.9	0
¼ t	Mustard	0	0	0
½ T	Brown Sugar	0	6.0	0
½ T	Worcestershire Sauce	0	0	0
½ C	Water	0	0	0
6 slices	Wheat Bread, Pepperidge Farm, light	12.0	42.0	2.0
2 t	Butter	0	0	7.2
		55.4	64.7	21.2
		7.9	7.1	7.0
		2.6	2.3	2.3

Brown ground beef with onions. Add remaining ingredients and heat. Divide into 3 sandwiches.

Grilled Ham and Cheese Sandwich

		P	C	F
2 slices	Wheat Bread, Pepperidge Farm, light	4.0	14.0	0.5
2 slices	American Cheese, reduced fat	8.0	4.0	6.0
½ T	Miracle Whip, fat free	0	1.0	0
1 slice	Cooked Ham, 96% extra lean	5.0	0	1.0
4	Pringles Fat Free Potato Chips	0.5	3.4	0
-	Salt and Pepper to taste	0	0	0
		17.5	22.4	7.5
		2.5	2.5	2.5

Turkey Salad Sandwich

		P	C	F
2 oz.	Turkey Breast, chopped (cooked)	13.5	0	0.8
2 slices	Wheat Bread, Pepperidge Farm, light	4.0	14.0	0.5
1 T	Miracle Whip, fat free	0	2.0	0
1 T	Miracle Whip, regular	0	2.0	7.0
1	Sweet Pickle, medium	0	8.0	0
		17.5	26.0	8.3
		2.5	2.8	2.7

Lunch - 2 Blocks

Chicken with Wild Rice Soup

		P	C	F
1 can	Chicken With Wild Rice	7.5	20.0	5.0
½	Hard Boiled Egg	3.0	0	2.5
1 slice	American Cheese, fat free	5.0	2.0	0
		18.5	22.0	7.5
		2.6	2.4	2.5

Beef with Vegetable & Barley Soup

		P	C	F
½ can	Beef With Vegetable & Barley	6.2	13.7	2.5
1	Hard Boiled Egg	6.0	0	5.0
½ oz.	Cheddar Cheese, reduced fat	4.0	0.5	0
1	Tangerine	0	9.0	0
		16.2	23.2	7.5
		2.3	2.5	2.5

Toasted Tomato Sandwich

		P	C	F
2 slices	Wheat Bread, Pepperidge Farm, light	4.0	14.0	0.5
1 T	Miracle Whip, regular	0	2.0	6.0
1 T	Miracle Whip, fat free	0	2.0	0
½	Tomato, medium	0.5	3.0	0
½ C	Cottage Cheese 2%	14.0	4.0	2.0
		18.5	24.0	8.5
		2.6	2.6	2.8

Chicken Noodle Soup

		P	C	F
1 can	Chicken Noodle	7.5	20.0	5.0
½	Hard Boiled Egg	3.0	0	2.5
1 slice	American Cheese, fat free	5.0	2.0	0
		15.5	22.0	7.5
		2.2	2.4	2.5

Vegetarian Vegetable Soup

		P	C	F
½ can	Vegetarian Vegetable	3.7	20.0	1.2
1	Hard Boiled Egg	6.0	0	5.0
1 slice	American Cheese, fat free	5.0	2.0	0
		14.7	22.0	6.2
		2.1	2.4	2.0

Lunch - 2 Blocks

Egg Salad Sandwich   P   C   F

		P	C	F
2 slices	Wheat Bread, Pepperidge Farm, light	4.0	14.0	0.5
1	Egg, Whole	6.0	0	5.0
1	Egg, White	4.0	0	0
2 T	Miracle Whip, fat free	0	4.0	0
½ t	Butter	0	0	1.8
5	Grapes	0	2.5	0
		14.0	20.5	7.3
		2.0	2.2	2.4

Minestrone Soup

		P	C	F
½ can	Minestrone	5.2	13.6	3.0
1 slice	Cooked Ham, 96% extra lean	5.0	0	1.0
1 slice	Wheat Bread, Pepperidge Farm, light	2.0	7.0	0
1 t	Butter	0	0	1.8
		12.2	20.6	5.8
		1.7	2.2	1.9

Chicken Noodle Soup with Chips

		P	C	F
1 can	Chicken Noodle	7.5	20.0	5.0
1	Hard Boiled Egg	6.0	0	5.0
1 oz.	Cheddar Cheese, fat free	8.0	1.0	0
4	Pringles Fat Free Potato Chips	0.5	4.0	0
		22.0	25.0	10.0
		3.1	2.7	3.3

B.L.T. with American Cheese

		P	C	F
2 slices	Wheat Bread, Pepperidge Farm, light	4.0	14.0	0.5
1½ slices	American Cheese, fat free	7.5	3.0	0
1 leaf	Romaine Lettuce	0	0	0
½	Tomato, medium	0.5	2.0	0
2½ slices	Bacon, lean	4.8	0	7.8
2 T	Miracle Whip, fat free	0	4.0	0
		16.8	23.0	8.3
		2.4	2.5	2.7

Lunch - 3 Blocks

Roast Beef Sandwich

		P	C	F
9 slices	Roast Beef, Deli-Thin 98% lean	14.6	2.5	1.0
2 slices	Wheat Bread, Pepperidge Farm, light	4.0	14.0	0.5
2	Lettuce Leaves	0	0	0
1 T	Horseradish	0	0	0
1 T	Miracle Whip, regular	0	2.0	7.0
8	Pringles Fat Free Potato Chips	1.0	6.8	0
1	Dill Pickle, medium	0	1.0	0
		19.6	27.3	8.5
		2.8	2.9	2.8

Ham & American Cheese Sandwich

		P	C	F
6 slices	Honey Ham, Deli-Thin 97% lean	10.0	2.0	1.5
2 slices	Wheat Bread, Pepperidge Farm, light	4.0	14.0	0.5
1 T	Miracle Whip, regular	0	2.0	7.0
1½ slices	American Cheese, fat free	7.5	3.0	0
1	Dill Pickle, medium	0	1.0	0
8	Pringles Fat Free Potato Chips	1.0	6.8	0
		22.5	28.8	9.0
		3.2	3.2	3.0

Hot Ham & Swiss

		P	C	F
2 slices	Wheat Bread, Pepperidge Farm, light	4.0	14.0	0.5
2 t	Butter	0	0	7.3
6 slices	Honey Ham, Deli-Thin 97% lean	10.0	2.0	1.5
1 slice	Swiss Cheese, fat free	8.0	1.0	0
1 slice	Onion, sliced thin	0	0	0
1 t	Horseradish	0	0	0
2 t	Mustard	0	0	0
1	Dill Pickle, medium	0	1.0	0
8	Pringles Fat Free Potato Chips	1.0	6.8	0
		23.0	24.8	9.8
		3.2	2.7	3.2

B.L.T. with Cheese

		P	C	F
2 slices	Wheat Bread, Pepperidge Farm, light	4.0	14.0	0.5
2 slice	American Cheese, fat free	10.0	4.0	0
1 leaf	Romaine Lettuce	0	0	0
½	Tomato, medium	0.5	2.0	0
3 slices	Bacon, lean	5.8	0	9.4
2 T	Miracle Whip, fat free	0	4.0	0
1	Sweet Pickle, small	0	4.0	0
		20.3	28.0	9.9
		2.9	3.1	3.3

Lunch - 3 Blocks

Chicken Noodle Soup and Ham Sandwich   P   C   F

		P	C	F
½ can	Chicken Noodle	3.7	10.0	2.5
6 slices	Honey Ham, Deli-Thin 97% lean	9.9	1.9	1.5
2 slices	Wheat Bread, Pepperidge Farm, light	4.0	14.0	0.5
½ t	Butter	0	0	1.8
½ T	Miracle Whip, regular	0	1.0	3.5
1	Lettuce Leaf, Romaine	0	0	0
1	American Cheese, fat free	5.0	2.0	0
4	Pringles Fat Free Potato Chips	0.5	3.4	0
		23.1	32.3	9.8
		3.3	3.5	3.3

Ham & Swiss Cheese Sandwich

		P	C	F
8 slices	Honey Ham, Deli-Thin 97% lean	13.3	2.6	2.0
2 slices	Wheat Bread, Pepperidge Farm, light	4.0	14.0	0.5
1 T	Miracle Whip, regular	0	2.0	7.0
1	Lettuce Leaf, Romaine	0	0	0
1	Swiss Cheese slice, fat free	5.0	3.0	0
2 t	Horseradish	0	2.0	0
6	Pringles Fat Free Potato chips	0.7	6.0	0
		22.7	29.6	9.5
		3.2	3.2	3.1

Ham & American Cheese Sandwich (Grapes)

		P	C	F
8 slices	Honey Ham, Deli-Thin 97% lean	13.3	2.6	2.0
2 slices	Wheat Bread, Pepperidge Farm, light	4.0	14.0	0.5
1 T	Miracle Whip, regular	0	2.0	7.0
1	Lettuce Leaf, Romaine	0	0	0
1	American Cheese, fat free	5.0	2.0	0
5	Grapes	0	2.5	0
8	Pringles Fat Free Potato Chips	1.0	6.8	0
		23.3	29.9	9.5
		3.3	3.3	3.1

Lunch - 3 Blocks

Ham & American Cheese Sandwich (Tangerine)

		P	C	F
8 slices	Honey Ham, Deli-Thin 97% lean	13.3	2.6	2.0
2 slices	Wheat Bread, Pepperidge Farm, light	4.0	14.0	0.5
1 T	Miracle Whip, regular	0	2.0	7.0
1	Lettuce Leaf, Romaine	0	0	0
1	American Cheese, fat free	5.0	2.0	0
1	Tangerine, small (2 oz. peeled weight)	0	7.0	0
4	Pringles Fat Free Potato Chips	0.5	3.4	0
		22.8	31.0	9.5
		3.2	3.4	3.1

Tuna Sandwich

		P	C	F
2.5 oz.	Tuna, Albacore, water packed	18.7	0	1.3
2 slices	Wheat Bread, Pepperidge Farm, light	4.0	14.0	0.5
2 T	Onion, diced	0	1.4	0.2
2	Lettuce Leaves	0	0	0
1 T	Miracle Whip, regular	0	2.0	7.0
1	Sweet Pickle, small	0	4.0	0
8	Pringles Fat Free Potato Chips	1.0	6.8	0
		23.7	28.2	9.3
		3.3	3.1	3.1

(9-oz. can of tuna makes 3 sandwiches)
(After draining, there is 7.5 oz of tuna.)

Tuna Melt

		P	C	F
2 oz.	Tuna, water packed	14.9	0	1.0
1 T	Green Onions, chopped	0.1	0.3	0
2 T	Miracle Whip, fat free	0	4.0	0
2 slices	Wheat Bread, Pepperidge Farm, light	4.0	14.0	0.5
1 slices	Swiss Cheese slice, regular	4.0	1.0	5.0
1 t	Butter	0	0	3.6
1	Sweet Pickle, small	0	4.0	0
6	Pringles Fat Free Potato Chips	0.7	6.0	0
2	Strawberry, large	0	1.0	0
		23.7	30.3	10.1
		3.3	3.3	3.3

Lunch - 3 Blocks

Beef with Vegetable and Barley and Tuna Sandwich

		P	C	F
½ Can	Beef With Vegetable & Barley Soup	6.2	11.2	2.5
2 slices	Wheat Bread, Pepperidge Farm, light	4.0	14.0	0.5
2 oz.	Tuna, albacore, water packed	13.0	0	1.0
2 T	Miracle Whip, fat free	0	4.0	0
1 T	Onions diced	.1	0.7	0
1½ t	Butter	0	0	5.4
		23.3	29.9	9.4
		3.3	3.3	3.1

Hot Pastrami

		P	C	F
6 slices	Pastrami, Deli-Thin 98% lean	11.0	1.0	1.0
2 slices	Rye Bread	4.0	22.0	2.0
1½ slices	Swiss Cheese, fat free	7.5	4.5	0
2 T	Mustard, Grey Poupon	0	0	0
2 slices	Onion, thin sliced	0	0	0
2 t	Butter	0	0	7.0
1	Dill Pickle, medium	0	1.0	0
		22.5	28.5	10.0
		3.2	3.1	3.3

Ready to Serve Chunky Beef Soup

		P	C	F
10.75 oz.	Chunky Beef Soup	15.0	24.0	5.0
12	Oyster Crackers	1.0	6.6	0.6
1	Hard Boiled Egg	6.0	0	5.0
		22.0	30.6	10.6
		3.1	3.4	3.5

Vegetarian Vegetable Soup & Ham Sandwich

		P	C	F
½ Can	Vegetarian Vegetable	3.7	20.0	1.2
2 slices	Wheat Bread, Pepperidge Farm, light	2.0	7.0	0
1½ slices	American Cheese, fat free	7.5	3.0	0
2 slices	Cooked Ham, 96% extra lean	10.0	0	3.0
1 T	Miracle Whip, regular	0	2.0	7.0
-	Salt and Pepper to taste	0	0	0
		23.2	32.0	11.2
		3.3	3.5	3.7

Lunch - 4 Blocks

Vegetarian Vegetable and
Grilled Ham and Cheese Sandwich   P   C   F

		P	C	F
½ can	Vegetarian Vegetable	3.7	20.0	1.2
2 slices	Wheat Bread, Pepperidge Farm, light	4.0	14.0	0.5
2 slices	American Cheese, reduced fat	8.0	4.0	6.0
1 t	Butter	0	0	3.6
½ T	Miracle Whip, fat free	0	1.0	0
2 slices	Cooked Ham, 96% extra lean	10.0	0	2.0
-	Salt and Pepper to taste	0	0	0
		25.7	39.0	13.3
		3.7	4.3	4.4

Ham and Swiss Cheese Sandwich 1½ Sandwiches

		P	C	F
9 slices	Honey Ham, Deli-Thin 97% lean	14.8	2.8	2.2
3 slices	Wheat Bread, Pepperidge Farm, light	6.0	22.0	1.0
1 t	Butter	0	0	3.6
1 T	Miracle Whip, regular	0	2.0	6.0
1	Lettuce Leaf, Romaine	0	0	0
1½	Swiss Cheese slice, fat free	7.5	4.5	0
1 t	Horseradish	0	1.0	0
5	Grapes	0	2.5	0
6	Pringles Fat Free Potato Chips	0.7	6.0	0
		29.0	40.8	12.8
		4.1	4.5	4.2

Chicken Noodle Soup and Turkey Salad Sandwich

		P	C	F
1 can	Chicken Noodle	3.7	10.0	2.5
3 oz.	Turkey Breast, chopped	20.2	0	1.2
2 slices	Wheat Bread, Pepperidge Farm, light	4.0	14.0	0.5
1 T	Miracle Whip, regular	0	2.0	7.0
1 T	Miracle Whip, fat free	0	2.0	0
1	Sweet Pickle, medium	0	8.0	0
		27.9	36.0	11.2
		3.9	4.0	3.7

Lunch - 4 Blocks

Ham Sandwiches (1½) & Tangerine

		P	C	F
9 slices	Honey Ham, Deli-Thin 97% lean	14.8	2.8	2.2
3 slices	Wheat Bread, Pepperidge Farm, light	6.0	22.0	1.0
1 t	Butter	0	0	3.6
1 T	Miracle Whip, regular	0	2.0	6.0
1	Lettuce Leaf, Romaine	0	0	0
1½	American Cheese, fat free	7.5	3.0	0
2 oz.	Tangerine, small (peeled weight)	0	7.0	0
4	Pringles Fat Free Potato Chips	0.5	3.4	0
		28.8	40.2	12.8
		4.1	4.4	4.2

Ham Sandwich 1½ Sandwiches & Grapes

		P	C	F
9 slices	Honey Ham, Deli-Thin 97% lean	14.8	2.8	2.2
3 slices	Wheat Bread, Pepperidge Farm, light	6.0	22.0	1.0
1 t	Butter	0	0	3.6
1 T	Miracle Whip, regular	0	2.0	6.0
1	Lettuce Leaf, Romaine	0	0	0
1½	American Cheese, fat free	7.5	3.0	0
10	Grapes	0	5.0	0
4	Pringles Fat Free Potato Chips	0.5	3.4	0
		28.8	38.2	12.8
		4.1	4.2	4.2

Patty Melt with Ground Beef and Smothered Onions

		P	C	F
3 oz.	Ground Beef 93% lean	15.7	0	4.5
1 slice	Swiss Cheese, fat free	5.0	3.0	0
2 slices	Wheat Bread, Pepperidge Farm, light	4.0	14.0	0.5
2 T	Mustard	0	0	0
-	Salt and Pepper to taste	0	0	0

Smothered Onions

		P	C	F
1 t	Vegetable Oil	0	0	4.6
½	Onion, medium, thinly sliced	0.4	2.8	0
-	Salt and Pepper to taste	0	0	0
8	Pringles Fat Free Potato Chips	1.0	8.0	0
1	Dill Pickle, medium	0	1.0	0
		31.4	38.8	12.6
		4.4	4.3	4.2

Lunch - 4 Blocks

Grilled Parmesan Beef Burger

		P	C	F
4 oz.	Ground Beef, 93%	21.0	0	6.0
2 t	Parmesan Cheese, regular, grated	2.0	0	1.5
1 t	Green Onions, chopped	0	0	0
-	Salt and Pepper to taste	0	0	0
2 slices	Wheat Bread, Pepperidge Farm, light	4.0	14.0	0.5
1 t	Butter	0	0	3.6
3	Onion Rings	0	0	0
8	Pringles Fat Free Potato Chips	1.0	8.0	0
2	Sweet Pickles, medium	0	16.0	0
		28.0	38.0	11.6
		4.0	4.2	3.8

Southwestern Cheeseburger

		P	C	F
3 oz.	Ground Beef 93%	15.7	0	4.5
1 T	Onions, finely chopped	0	0	0
2 T	Green Chili's, diced	0	1.0	0
1 slice	Monterey Jack Cheese, light	9.0	0.3	6.0
1	Kaiser Roll	2.8	14.9	1.2
4 T	Pace Salsa	0	6.0	0
8	Pringles Fat Free Potato Chips	1.0	8.0	0
1	Sweet Pickle, medium	1.0	8.0	0
		29.5	35.2	11.7
		4.2	3.9	3.9

Grilled Parmesan Turkey Burger

		P	C	F
3 oz.	Ground Turkey Breast, skinless	20.2	0	1.2
2 T	Parmesan Cheese, fat free, grated	3.0	9.0	0
1 t	Green Onions, chopped	0	0	0
-	Salt and Pepper to taste	0	0	0
1	Hamburger Bun	4.0	22.0	1.0
1 T	Butter	0	0	11.0
3	Onion Rings, raw	0	0	0
8	Pringles Fat Free Potato Chips	1.0	8.0	0
		28.8	39.0	13.1
		4.1	4.3	4.3

Lunch - 4 Blocks

Reuben Sandwich		P	C	F
12 slices	Corned Beef, Deli Thin, lean	14.0	1.0	5.0
2 slices	Pumpernickel Bread	6.0	23.6	2.0
1½ slice	Swiss Cheese, fat free	7.5	4.5	0
¼ C	Sauerkraut	0	2.0	0
1½ T	Thousand Island Dressing, regular	0	3.7	5.0
1 T	Miracle Whip, fat free	0	2.0	0
1	Dill Pickle, medium	0	1.0	0
	27.5	37.8	12.0
	3.9	4.2	4.0

Patty Melt with Ground Turkey and Smothered Onions		P	C	F
3 oz.	Ground Turkey Breast, skinless	20.2	0	1.2
1/8 t	Thyme Leaves, dried	0	0	0
1/8 t	Oregano, dried	0	0	0
1	Garlic Clove, small	0	0	0
1 slice	Swiss Cheese, fat free	5.0	3.0	0
2 slices	Rye Bread	4.2	22.0	2.0
2 T	Mustard	0	0	0
-	Salt and Pepper	0	0	0
8	Pringles Fat Free Potato Chips	1.0	8.0	0
1	Sweet Pickle, medium	0	8.0	0

Smothered Onions
2 t | Vegetable Oil | 0 | 0 | 9.2
½ | Onion, medium, thinly sliced | 0 | 3.0 | 0
1/8 t | Salt | 0 | 0 | 0
- | Pepper | 0 | 0 | 0
| | 30.4 | 41.0 | 12.4
| | 4.3 | 4.5 | 4.1

Beef Dinner Choices

Dinner - 4 Blocks

Braised Beef with Vegetable and Barley for 3		**P**	**C**	**F**
12 oz	Bottom Round Steak, trimmed	80.2	0	12.2
2½ T	Butter	0	0	27.5
½ C	Onions, chopped	0.9	5.6	0.1
1 C	Mushrooms, sliced	2.0	2.2	0.4
2	Garlic Cloves, minced	0	0	0
1 can	Beef Broth	0	0	0
1	Bay Leaf	0	0	0
-	Salt and Pepper to taste	0	0	0
1 C	Frozen Peas	7.7	12.0	0.4
4 T	Sour Cream, fat free	6.0	1.2	0
3 T	Pearl Barley	1.9	20.6	0.3
5	Potatoes, New Red, 2.5" (10 oz.)	5.2	37.2	0
1 C	Carrots, diced	2.0	23.0	0
3	Peaches	0	27.0	0
		104.0	128.8	40.9
		14.8	14.3	13.6
		4.9	4.7	4.5

Place the butter in a Dutch oven or a skillet and brown the beef over medium heat. Remove the beef and set aside.

Add the onions, mushrooms, and garlic to the skillet and sauté until tender. Return the beef to the skillet, add broth, bay leaf, salt and pepper and bring to a boil. Reduce heat, cover and simmer for about an hour.

Add the barley, cover and simmer for another 45 minutes or until the beef and barley are tender.

Add the peas, cover and simmer until peas are tender. (About 5 minutes.)

Discard bay leaf. Cut beef into 3 equal pieces and put on plates. Cover with the barley gravy and serve. Eat a peach for dessert. You can substitute another fruit for the peaches.

Divide and weigh each meal to assure the meals all weigh the same, within a few tenths of an ounce.

Dinner - 5 Blocks

Beef Stroganoff for 3   P   C   F

		P	C	F
10 oz.	Top Sirloin Steak	86.0	0	19.2
2 C	Onions, diced	3.6	22.4	0.4
-	Fat Free Cooking Spray	0	0	0
2 T	Butter	0	0	22.0
-	Salt and Pepper to taste	0	0	0
4.5 oz. can	Mushrooms, with juice	1.0	2.0	0
1	Beef Bouillon Cube	0	1.0	0
2 T	Cornstarch	0	14.0	0
1½ C	Water	0	0	0
½ C	Sour Cream, fat free	8.0	16.0	0
3 oz.	Egg Noodles, 2 C dry	8.0	38.0	2.4

Mandarin Orange Salad:

		P	C	F
2 C	Romaine Lettuce	6.0	10.0	0
27	Grapes	0	12.5	0
1½ C	Strawberries, sliced	1.5	10.5	0
1 C	Mandarin Oranges, light	1.0	16.0	0
1 T	Mandarin Orange Salad Dressing	0	3.0	1.1
		115.1	145.4	45.1
		16.4	16.1	15.0
		5.4	5.3	5.0

Mandarin Orange Salad Dressing: (Makes 4 Tablespoons.)
- 1 t   Canola Oil
- 3 T   Mandarin Orange liquid, light
- 1 t   Red Wine Vinegar
- 1 t   Cider Vinegar
- 1 t   Sugar

    Cook noodles according to the package directions and set aside. (Run hot water over the noodles to reheat when ready to serve.)

    Cut Steak into thin strips. Spray a cool skillet with a fat free cooking spray. Add butter and heat. Add meat strips and onions and brown. (About 10 minutes.) Add beef bouillon cube, salt, pepper, ½ Cup of water and liquid from the canned mushrooms. Bring to a boil, reduce heat to low, cover and simmer about ½ hour, or until meat is fork tender.

    Add the mushrooms and heat. Remove beef mixture to a warm plate. Keep warm.

    Stir the cornstarch and 1½ Cups of water together and gradually add to the skillet. Cook over medium heat until the sauce thickens. Stir in the sour cream. Heat thoroughly but do not boil. Return beef to the skillet and stir, making sure to coat beef completely. Divide the noodles and beef. Spoon the beef mixture over the noodles and serve.

    Combine salad dressing ingredients, shake well and pour 1 Tablespoons over the lettuce. Mix well, divide and place in bowls. Cut Grapes in half. Divide mandarin oranges, strawberries and grapes. Place on top of the lettuce. (You can omit the strawberries, grapes or mandarin oranges and still have a balanced meal.) Divide and weigh each meal to assure the meals all weigh the same within a few tenths of an ounce.

    Divide and weigh each meal to assure the meals all weigh the same, within a few tenths of an ounce.

Dinner - 4 Blocks

Meat Loaf for 3		P	C	F
14 oz.	Ground Beef, 93% lean	73.5	0	21.0
2 slices	Wheat Bread, Pepperidge Farm, light	4.0	14.0	0.5
½ C	Onions, diced	0.4	2.8	0
¼ C	Green Pepper, diced	0.1	1.4	0
1	Egg	4.0	0	5.0
-	Fat Free Cooking Spray	0	0	0
9 T	Heinz Ketchup	0	36.0	0
1½ C	Cauliflower	3.0	7.5	0
1 Can	Asparagus	7.0	7.0	0
1½ T	Butter	0	0	16.5
Dessert:				
3 C	Strawberries, sliced	3.0	21.0	0
¾ C	Cool Whip, fat free	0	18.0	0
1 T	Sugar	0	12.0	0
		95.0	119.7	43.0
		13.5	13.3	14.3
		4.5	4.4	4.7

Place ground beef in a large bowl. Mix in the bread crumbs, onions, green pepper, and egg white. Blend well and shape in a loaf pan. Bake in a 350-degree oven for about 1 hour, or until the meatloaf is no longer pink.

Steam cauliflower. Heat asparagus. Divide butter in half and melt over each of the vegetables.

(You can omit the strawberries and sugar and fat free whipped topping, And Add 3 slices of Wheat Bread, light, minus the butter, and 6 more tablespoons of ketchup and you will still be eating a 4 block meal. Or try another substitution.)

Divide and weigh each meal to assure the meals all weigh the same, within a few tenths of an ounce.

Dinner - 4 Blocks

Beef Stew for 4		**P**	**C**	**F**
16 oz.	Bottom Round, lean	107.5	0	17.2
5 T	Flour	3.7	27.5	0
-	Fat Free Cooking Spray	0	0	0
2 T	Canola Oil	0	0	28.0
¾ C	Onions, chopped	1.5	8.4	0
1	Garlic Clove, minced	0	0	0
1 t	Worcestershire Sauce	0	0	0
3 C	Water	0	0	0
-	½ t Salt, ¼ t Pepper	0	0	0
2	Beef Bouillon Cubes	0	2.0	0
10	Potatoes, New Red, 2.5" (20 oz.)	6.6	46.6	0
1 C	Carrots, diced	2.0	23.0	0
1 C	Peas, frozen	8.0	18.0	0
8 slices	Wheat Bread, Pepperidge Farm, light	18.6	58.6	2.6
1½ T	Butter	0	0	16.5
		147.9	184.1	64.3
		21.1	20.4	21.4
		5.2	5.1	5.3

Cut beef into 1 to 1½" pieces. Coat meat with flour. Shake off excess flour and reserve. Spray a Dutch oven with fat free cooking spray, add the oil, and brown the meat all over, a few pieces at a time, removing them as they brown.

Reduce heat to medium. To the drippings in pan, add onions and garlic. Cook 3 minutes, stirring until onions are almost tender. Stir in reserve flour. Combine Worcestershire Sauce, Beef Bouillon Cube, Water, and the Salt and Pepper. Gradually add to mixture in the pan. Cook, stirring, until slightly thickened.

Return the meat to the pan and bring to a boil, stirring. Reduce heat to low, cover, and simmer for 2½ hours, or until the meat is tender, stirring occasionally.

Add potatoes and carrots. Bring to a boil, reduce heat to low, cover and simmer another 20 minutes. Add the peas, cover and simmer until vegetables and meat are tender. Serve two slices of bread per person.

Makes about 5 cups of beef stew. Serves about 1 ¼ C of beef stew with 2 slices of bread per person.

Divide and weigh each meal to assure the meals all weigh the same, within a few tenths of an ounce.

Dinner - 4 Blocks

Spaghetti for 6

Amount	Ingredient	P	C	F
20 oz.	Ground Beef, 93%	105.0	0	30.0
½ C	Onions, diced	0.9	5.6	0.1
28 oz.	Whole Tomatoes	7.0	21.0	0
45 oz.	Tomato Sauce	21.0	42.0	0
1 T	Brown Sugar	0	12.0	0
2½ T	Oregano	0	0	0
¼ C	Parsley Flakes	0	0	0
½ t	Garlic, granulated	0	0	0
1/8 t	Thyme	0	0	0
1	Bay Leaf	0	0	0
6 oz.	Angel Hair Spaghetti	21.0	120.0	3.0
6 T	Parmesan Cheese, grated, regular	18.0	0	13.8
6 slices	Wheat Bread, Pepperidge Farm, light	14.0	44.0	2.0
½ t	Garlic, granulated	0	0	0
3 T	Butter	0	0	33.0
		186.9	244.6	81.9
		26.7	27.1	27.3
		4.4	4.5	4.5

Makes about ¾ C each serving.

Brown meat and onions in skillet. Add the next 7 ingredients, and simmer about 2 hours, or until sauce is thick. Cook the 6-oz. spaghetti. (Use spices to suit your own taste.)

Divide and weigh the cooked spaghetti and place on 6 plates. Discard Bay Leaf. Pour ¾ C (1/6 Th of the sauce) over the spaghetti. Sprinkle 1 Tablespoon of Parmesan cheese over the sauce.

Toast bread. Stir garlic powder into the butter and spread ½ Tablespoon on each piece of toast. Place the garlic-buttered toast under the broiler just until the butter starts to bubble. Serve one slice of garlic toast with each meal.

Divide and weigh each meal to assure the meals all weigh the same, within a few tenths of an ounce.

Dinner - 4 Blocks

Pepper Steak Stir-Fry for 3		P	C	F
9 oz.	Flank Steak	68.8	0	25.5
2	Garlic Cloves, minced	0	0	0
1 T	Olive Oil	0	0	14.0
-	Fat Free Cooking Spray	0	0	0
½ C	Beef Broth	0	0	0
½ t	Ginger Root, grated	0	0	0
1 T	Corn Starch	0	7.0	0
¾ C	Green Pepper, 1" squares	0.6	7.8	0.1
¾ C	Onion, 1" squares	1.3	7.8	0.1
1 C	Cauliflower, raw	2.0	5.0	0
1 C	Broccoli, raw	3.0	6.0	0.5
4 T	Soy Sauce	4.0	4.0	0
¼ C	White Rice, raw (1 Cup cooked)	4.0	38.0	0
Dessert:				
2 C	Strawberries	2.0	14.0	0
12 T	Cool Whip, fat free	0	18.0	0
		85.7	107.6	40.2
		12.2	11.9	13.4
		4.0	3.9	4.4

Prepare rice as directed on package but omit the butter. (Covered and set aside.)

In a small bowl, combine beef broth, gingerroot, and cornstarch. Mix well. Set aside.

Cut beef lengthwise into thin strips. Spray wok with fat free cooking spray; add oil and heat over medium high heat. Add beef and garlic. Cook, stirring, about 3 minutes, or until beef is browned. Remove beef from wok, cover and keep warm.

Reduce heat to medium; add green peppers, onions, cauliflower, and broccoli. Cook and stir 5 to 7 minutes, or until vegetables are crisp-tender. Add soy sauce. Stir the cornstarch mixture until it's smooth. Add to the wok. Cook, stirring 2 to 3 minutes more, until sauce is thickened and bubbly. Divide vegetables by 3. (You don't have to worry too much about dividing each individual vegetable evenly as they are just about the same PFC's.)

Divide beef into 3, making sure they all weigh about the same, return beef to wok, cook until thoroughly heated. (To make it easier when you return the beef to the wok, place each serving in separate sections.) Place 1/3 cup of warm rice on each plate and add the divided beef and vegetables.

(You can omit the strawberries and fat free whipped topping, and add another 1/2 C of cooked rice, and the meal will be balanced.)

Divide and weigh each meal to assure the meals all weigh the same, within a few tenths of an ounce.

Dinner - 4 Blocks

Beef Top Round with Horseradish Sauce for 3   P   C   F

		P	C	F
12 oz.	Beef Top Round (4 oz. each)	73.9	0	12.7
1 T	Flour	0.7	5.5	0
-	Fat Free Cooking Spray	0	0	0
2 T	Butter	0	0	22.0
1	Garlic Clove, minced	0	0	0
1	Bay Leaf	0	0	0
2 t	Worcestershire Sauce	0	0	0
½ t	Marjoram, dried	0	0	0
-	Salt and Pepper to taste	0	0	0
8	Potatoes, Red small chunks (16 oz.)	5.3	37.3	0
¾ C	Carrots, cut in chunks	1.5	17.2	0
½ C	Onions, chopped	0.4	2.8	0

Horseradish Cream Sauce:

		P	C	F
¾ C	Milk 2%	6.0	8.2	3.7
1 T	Cornstarch	0	9.0	0
1 t	Mustard, Grey Poupon	0	0	0
-	Salt to taste	0	0	0

Mandarin Orange Salad:

		P	C	F
3 C	Romaine Lettuce	9.0	15.0	0
15	Grapes	0	7.5	0
¼ C	Mandarin Oranges, light	0.5	8.0	0
2 T	Mandarin Orange Salad Dressing	0	6.0	1.1
		97.3	116.5	39.5
		13.9	12.9	13.1
		4.6	4.3	4.3

Mandarin Orange Salad Dressing:

1 t	Canola Oil
3 T	Mandarin Orange liquid, light
1 t	Red Wine Vinegar
1 t	Cider Vinegar
1 t	Sugar

    Spray a cool skillet with non-stick spray; add the butter and heat. Coat the beef with flour and brown. Remove beef from skillet and put in a casserole dish. Add a small amount of water and the next 6 ingredients.

    Bake at 350 degrees for about 1 hours, or until the beef is tender, adding more water as necessary. Add the vegetables and continue baking until they are tender. Serve horseradish cream sauce on the side.

    Combine salad dressing ingredients, shake well and pour 2 Tablespoons over the lettuce. Mix well, divide and place in bowls. Cut grapes in half. Divide mandarin oranges and grapes and place on top of the lettuce. (You can omit the grapes or mandarin oranges and still have a balanced meal.)

    Divide and weigh beef, potatoes and carrots (within a few 10th of an oz.) to assure the meals all have the same amount of each.

Dinner - 4 Blocks

Beef Top Round with Vegetables for 3		P	C	F
12 oz.	Beef Top Round	73.9	0	12.7
2 T	Flour	1.4	11.0	0
-	Fat Free Cooking Spray	0	0	0
7 t	Butter	0	0	25.6
2	Black Peppercorns, whole	0	0	0
1	Garlic Clove, minced	0	0	0
2 t	Worcestershire Sauce	0	0	0
1 C	Red Wine	0	0	0
1 T	Parsley	0	0	0
-	Salt and Pepper to taste	0	0	0
9	Potatoes, Red small chunks (18 oz.)	6.0	42.0	0
1 Can	Green Beans	1.0	13.5	0
½ C	Onions, chopped	0.4	2.8	0

Mandarin Orange Salad:				
4 C	Romaine Lettuce	12.0	20.0	0
¼ C	Mandarin Oranges, light	0.5	8.0	0
15	Grapes	0	7.5	0
2 T	Mandarin Orange Salad Dressing	0	6.0	2.2
		95.2	110.8	40.5
		13.6	12.3	13.5
		4.5	4.1	4.5

Mandarin Orange Salad Dressing:
1 t	Canola Oil
3 T	Mandarin Orange liquid, light
1 t	Red Wine Vinegar
1 t	Cider Vinegar
1 t	Sugar

Spray a cool skillet with fat free cooking spray; add the butter and heat. Coat the beef with flour and brown. Remove beef from skillet and put in a casserole dish. Add a small amount of water and the next 6 ingredients.
Bake at 350 degrees for about 1 hours, or until the beef is tender, adding more water as necessary. Add the vegetables and continue baking until they are tender.

Combine salad dressing ingredients, shake well and pour 2 Tablespoons over the lettuce. Mix well, divide and place in bowls. Cut Grapes in half. Divide mandarin oranges and grapes. Place on top of the lettuce.

(You can omit the grapes or mandarin oranges and still have a balanced meal.)

Divide and weigh beef, potatoes and carrots (within a few 10th of an oz.) to assure the meals all have the same amount of each.

Dinner - 4 Blocks

Shredded Beef Chimichangas for 3

		P	C	F
8 oz.	Top Round Roast, lean	61.4	0	8.6
1	Beef Bouillon Cube	0	1.0	0
8 oz.	Pace Salsa	0	21.0	0
1 C	Refried Beans, fat free	14.0	22.0	0
6	Manny's Flour Tortillas, (6")	6.0	72.0	6.0
2 t	Taco Seasoning	0	3.4	0
2.5 oz.	Cheddar Cheese, regular, grated	17.5	2.5	22.5
8 oz.	Green Chiles, diced	1.0	8.0	0
		99.9	130.9	37.1
		14.2	14.5	12.3
		4.7	4.8	4.1

Preheat oven to 350 degrees.

Remove all visible fat from the top round roast. Put a little water in a small roasting pan, cover, and braise at 350 degree until beef shreds easily with a fork.

Place the shredded beef into a large bowl; add salsa, refried beans, taco seasoning, green chiles, and half the grated cheese. Stir until well blended.

The beef mixture should weigh about 26.5 ounces, making about 4.4 ounces of beef mixture for each tortilla.

Divide the meat mixture into 6 equal portions and place in the center of the flour tortillas. Roll the tortillas, place in a casserole dish and sprinkle the remaining cheese on top. Heat in the oven until the cheese is meat mixture is hot and the cheese is melted. (3 per person.)

If you would like to use the chimichangas as a 2-block snack, put all the cheese inside the tortillas and only eat one.

Divide and weigh each meal to assure the meals all weigh the same, within a few tenths of an ounce.

Dinner - 4 Blocks

Beef Burritos for 3

		P	C	F
12 oz.	Ground Beef, 93% lean	63.0	0	18.0
1 t	Butter	0	0	3.6
½ t	Taco Seasoning	0	0.8	0
4.5 oz.	Green Chiles, diced	0	4.0	0
½ C	Onions, diced	0.8	5.6	0
1 C	Refried Beans, fat free	14.0	22.0	0
1 oz.	Monterey Jack Cheese, reduced fat, grated	9.0	0.3	6.0
1½ oz.	Cheddar Cheese, reduced fat, grated	9.0	3.0	6.0
½ C	Lettuce, chopped finely	1.0	2.0	0
1 C	Tomatoes, diced	0	6.0	0
6	Manny's Flour Tortillas, (6")	6.0	72.0	6.0
5 oz.	Enchilada Sauce	0	6.7	1.7
		102.8	122.4	41.3
		14.6	13.6	13.7
		4.8	4.5	4.5

In a skillet, brown ground beef with butter. Add Taco Seasoning, diced green chiles, onions, refried beans, Monterey Jack Cheese and Cheddar Cheese. Heat until hot, stirring to melt cheese.

Add diced tomato and lettuce; stir just long enough to blend. Divide into 6 equal portions. (About 3.5 oz. each) Put on the tortillas, roll and place in the oven or microwave to heat. Heat the Enchilada Sauce. Divide and pour over the burrito. Two beef burrito's per person.

Divide and weigh each meal to assure the meals all weigh the same, within a few tenths of an ounce.

Dinner - 5 Blocks

Beef Fajitas for 3		P	C	F
10.5 oz.	Beef Top Round, lean	73.5	0	9.4
-	Fat Free Cooking Spray	0	0	0
1½ T	Olive Oil	0	0	21.0
1 T	Taco Seasoning	0	1.6	0
1 t	Chili Powder	0	0	0
¼ t	Cumin	0	0	0
1 t	Salt	0	0	0
1½ C	Onions, cut into strips	2.7	16.8	0.3
½ C	Green Pepper, cut into strips	0.7	5.6	0.2
½ C	Red Pepper, cut into strips	0.7	5.6	0.2
½ C	Tomatoes, diced	0	3.0	0
6	Manny's Tortilla's, (6")	6.0	72.0	6.0
3 t	Sour Cream, fat free	1.5	0.5	0
1 C	Refried Beans, fat free	14.0	22.0	0
1½ oz.	Cheddar Cheese, reduced fat, grated	9.0	3.0	6.0
6 T	Pace Salsa	0	6.0	0
		108.1	136.1	43.1
		15.5	15.1	14.3
		5.1	5.0	4.8

Slice the beef across the grain into thin strips. Combine chili powder, Taco seasoning, cumin and salt and stir into the beef strips, blend well. Dice the tomatoes and set aside.

Spray a skillet with fat free cooking spray and, over medium-high heat fry the onions and green peppers until crisp-tender and brown in spots.

Meanwhile spray another skillet with fat free cooking spray; add the olive oil and heat. Add the strips to the skillet. Cook over medium high heat for 2 to 3 minutes or until brown and tender.

Heat tortilla's, one at a time in a skillet. (Heating in microwave may make the tortillas rubbery.) Heat the refried beans; divide by 3, spread over the warm tortillas. Divide sour cream, tomatoes, meat, cheeses and vegetables into 3 equal servings. Use 1 Tablespoons of salsa and ½ t sour cream on each fajita. Serves 3 people 2 Fajitas each.

Divide and weigh each meal to assure the meals all weigh the same, within a few tenths of an ounce.

Dinner - 5 Blocks

Minnesota Taco's for 3

		P	C	F
10 oz.	Ground Beef, 93% lean	52.4	0	15.0
15 oz.	Tomato Sauce	2.0	14.0	0
1 C	Canned Chili with beans	15.0	14.0	9.0
½ C	Open Pit Original B.B.Q. Sauce	0	44.0	2.0
1 C	Cheddar Cheese, reduced fat, grated	8.0	2.6	5.3
½ C	Onions, diced	0.8	5.4	0
½ C	Green Pepper, diced	0.4	5.4	0
1 C	Lettuce, shredded	1.3	2.7	0
1	Tomatoes, medium	2.0	6.0	0

Tortillas: Makes 3 large tortillas

3 T	Flour, White	2.0	16.2	0.1
3 T	Corn Meal, yellow	2.0	19.0	0.5
1 T	Corn Starch	0	7.0	0
½ t	Salt	0	0	0
1	Egg, whole	6.0	0	5.0
½ C	Milk, 2%	4.0	6.0	2.5
½ T	Canola Oil	0	0	7.0
-	Non-Stick Spray	0	0	0
		95.9	142.3	46.4
		13.7	15.8	15.4
		4.5	5.2	5.1

Brown ground beef in an electric skillet. Stir in tomato sauce and chili without beans. Keep warm.

Mix all the ingredients for tortillas. Spray a large skillet with non-stick spray and heat. Pour 1/3 rd of the tortilla mixture onto the heated skillet. Gently turn the skillet to spread the batter, making it as large and thin as possible. Makes 3 tortilla's. Place the tortillas in a pre-warmed oven to keep warm.

Dice the onions, tomatoes and green peppers, divide by 3 and place into 3 individual bowls. Shred the lettuce; divide by 3 and place on top of the vegetables. Grate the cheese; divide by 3 and place on top of the shredded lettuce. Divide the B.B.Q. Sauce by 3. (When you are ready to make them it won't make any difference how much you put on each tortilla, just as long as they are equally divided by 3 before placing in the bowls.) Divide the ground beef mixture by 3.

Put 1/3rd of the meat mixture in the middle of each tortilla; sprinkle on 1/2 of the diced vegetables. Top with 1/2 of the B.B.Q. Sauce. Fold up the bottom flap and then fold sides over diaper style. Makes 2 Tortilla's per person.

Divide and weigh each meal to assure the meals all weigh the same, within a few tenths of an ounce.

Dinner -4 Blocks

Texas Hash for 4

16 oz.	Ground Beef, 93% lean	84.0	0	24.0
¼ C	Onions, diced	0.4	2.8	0
¼ C	Green Pepper, diced	0.2	2.8	0
28 oz.	Whole Tomatoes, canned	7.0	21.0	0
15 oz.	Tomato Sauce	7.0	21.0	0
-	Salt and Pepper to taste	0	0	0
1/3 C	White Rice, uncooked	5.3	50.6	0
8 slices	Wheat Bread, Pepperidge Farm, light	16.0	64.0	2.6
2½ T	Butter (1 t per slice)	0	0	27.5
		119.9	146.2	54.1
		17.1	18.0	18.0
		4.2	4.5	4.5

Brown ground beef with diced onions and green pepper. Add whole tomatoes and tomato sauce. Season with salt and pepper to taste. Rinse cans out with about 1-Cup water and add to the mixture along with the uncooked rice. Cook for 20 minutes, stirring often to keep from sticking. Makes about 1 3/4 Cups of Texas Hash per person. Serve with 2 slices of bread each person.

Divide and weigh each meal to assure the meals all weigh the same, within a few tenths of an ounce.

Dinner - 5 Blocks

Lasagna for 6			P	C	F
16 oz.	Ground Beef 93%		84.0	0	24.0
½ C	Onions, diced		0.9	5.6	0.1
2	Garlic Cloves		0	0	0
1 T	Brown Sugar		0	12.0	0
2 T	Oregano		0	0	0
1/8 t	Thyme		0	0	0
¼ C	Parsley Flakes		0	0	0
1	Bay Leaf		0	0	0
28 oz.	Whole Tomatoes		7.0	21.0	0
45 oz.	Tomato Sauce		21.0	42.0	0
8 oz.	Mozzarella Cheese, reduced fat		72.0	8.0	16.0
4.5 oz.	Lasagna Noodles (6)		15.7	90.0	2.2
12 slices	Wheat Bread, Pepperidge Farm, light		28.0	88.0	4.0
4½ T	Butter		0	0	49.5
½ t	Garlic, Granulated		0	0	0
			228.6	266.6	95.8
			32.6	29.6	31.9
			5.4	4.9	5.3

Heat oven to 350 degrees.

Brown meat, onions and garlic in skillet. Add the next 7 ingredients and simmer about 2 hours or until sauce is thick. (Use spices to suit your own taste.) Discard Bay Leaf.

Cook lasagna noodles. Slice the cheese in 24 fairly equal pieces, weigh and divide into 6 equal portions. (About 1.4 oz. on each layer of the 6 portions.) Cover the bottom of a rectangle casserole dish with a thin layer of sauce. Place 3 lasagna noodles on sauce. Divide the rest of the sauce in about half. Put one half the sauce and half the cheese on top of the sauce. Add the rest of the noodles, top with the remaining sauce and cheese. (12 slices of cheese per layer. 4 slices of cheese per serving.)
Bake for about 20 minutes or until the cheese is melted.

While the lasagna is baking, toast 12 slices of bread. (or 2 for each person.) Stir garlic powder into the butter and spread on the toast.

Remove the lasagna pan from the oven and let stand for about 10 minutes before serving.
Divide the lasagna into six portions. If all the lasagna is not served at the meal freeze in individual containers for future meal or serve for dinner tomorrow night.

Divide and weigh each meal to assure the meals all weigh the same, within a few tenths of an ounce.

Dinner - 4 Blocks

Steak and Potatoes for 3   P   C   F

		P	C	F
9 oz.	Top Sirloin, lean (3 oz. each)	77.4	0	17.3
3 T	Worcestershire Sauce	0	0	0
½ t	Onion Salt	0	0	0
½ t	Garlic Powder	0	0	0
1 t	Meat Tenderizer	0	0	0
7	Potatoes, Red small chunks (14 oz.)	4.6	32.6	0
1 C	Broccoli	3.0	6.0	0.5
1 C	Carrots, cut in chunks	2.0	23.0	0
2 T	Butter	0	0	22.0

Mandarin Orange Salad:

		P	C	F
2 C	Romaine Lettuce	6.0	10.0	0
¼ C	Mandarin Oranges, light	0.5	8.0	0
20	Grapes	0	10.0	0
1½ C	Strawberries, sliced	1.5	14.0	0
2 t	Sugar	0	8.0	0
2 T	Mandarin Orange Salad Dressing	0	6.0	2.2
		95.0	117.6	42.0
		13.5	13.0	14.0
		4.5	4.3	4.6

Mandarin Orange Salad Dressing:

1 t	Canola Oil
3 T	Mandarin Orange liquid, light
1 t	Red Wine Vinegar
1 t	Cider Vinegar
1 t	Sugar

Cut all visible fat from the steak and weigh. Cut into 3 equal pieces, 3 oz. each. Sprinkle meat tenderizer, garlic powder, and onion salt. Rub into meat. Using a fork, stab the spices deep into the meat. Pour Worcestershire sauce on each piece and stab again. Grill the meat.

Steam the potatoes, broccoli and carrots in separate sides of the steamer. (Making it easier to divide when ready to serve. Melt the butter over the steamed vegetables and serve.

Combine salad dressing ingredients, shake well and pour 2 Tablespoons over the lettuce. Mix well, divide and place in bowls. Cut Grapes in half. Dice the strawberries, put 2t sugar on them and mix well. Divide mandarin oranges, strawberries and grapes. Place on top of the lettuce.

(You can omit the grapes or mandarin oranges and still have a balanced meal.)

Divide and weigh beef. Weigh the potatoes, broccoli and carrots, divide and serve, (within a few 10th of an oz,) to assure the meals all have the same amount of each.

Dinner - 5 Blocks

Veal Scaloppini for 3		P	C	F
12 oz.	Veal Cutlets (3.5 oz. each)	90.1	0	20.9
1 T	Flour	0.7	5.5	0
-	Fat Free Cooking Spray	0	0	0
8 oz.	Red Wine	0	0	0
-	Salt and Pepper to taste	0	0	0
4	Red Potatoes, small (8 oz.)	2.6	18.6	0
1 C	Broccoli	3.0	6.0	0.5
7 t	Butter	0	0	25.2
Dessert:				
3 slices	1/12th Angel Food Cake	9.0	90.0	0
1½ C	Strawberries, sliced	1.5	10.5	0
6 T	Cool Whip, fat free	0	9.0	0
		106.9	139.6	46.6
		15.2	15.5	15.5
		5.0	5.1	5.1

Follow angel food cake directions. When baked, slice into 12 fairly equal pieces.

Place veal between 2 pieces of wax paper and pound lightly. Make small incisions around the edges of the cutlets to prevent them from rolling while they cook. Coat veal with flour. Shake off excess.

Spray a cool skillet with fat free cooking spray. Arrange cutlets in the skillet so that they don't touch each other. Sauté over medium heat until brown. (About 3 minutes) Transfer cutlets to a heated plate. Keep warm.

Add wine to the skillet, scrape up all the particles add salt and pepper to taste. Bring to a boil. Pour evenly over the cutlets. Serve immediately.

Steam vegetables and melt the butter over them.

Serve angel food cake with a fat free Cool Whip and strawberries for dessert. (You can omit the strawberries and still have a balanced meal.)

Divide and weigh each meal to assure the meals all weigh the same, within a few tenths of an ounce.

Dinner - 4 Blocks

Veal with Vegetables and Gravy for 3

		P	C	F
9 oz.	Veal Cutlets (3 oz. each)	67.5	0	15.6
2 T	Flour, white	1.5	11.0	0
½ T	Canola Oil	0	0	7.0
-	Fat Free Cooking Spray	0	0	0
1 C	Carrots, sliced	2.0	23.0	0
6	Potatoes, New Red, small (12 oz.)	4.0	27.8	0
½ C	Onions, chopped	0.9	5.6	0.1
1	Celery Stalk, chopped	0	2.0	0
1 T	Butter	0	0	11.0
1 C	White Wine	0	0	0
1 C	Water	0	0	0
1 t	Parsley, dried	0	0	0
3 C	Romaine Lettuce	9.0	15.0	0
¼ C	Mandarin Oranges	0.5	8.0	0
1 C	Strawberries, sliced	1.0	7.0	0
10	Grapes	0	5.0	0
2 T	Mandarin Orange Salad Dressing	0	6.0	2.2
		86.4	110.4	35.9
		12.3	12.2	11.9
		4.1	4.0	3.9

Mandarin Orange Salad Dressing

1 t	Canola Oil
3 T	Mandarin Orange liquid, light
1 t	Red Wine Vinegar
1 t	Cider Vinegar
1 t	Sugar

Place veal between 2 pieces of wax paper and pound lightly. Make small incisions around the edges of the cutlets to prevent them from rolling while they cook. Coat veal with flour. Shake off excess.

Spray skillet with fat free cooking spray; add the oil and heat. Add the onions, carrots and celery. Cook over medium heat for 3 minutes, stirring frequently. Add the veal and brown on all sides. Mix together the wine, water and flour. Add to the skillet. Make sure the meat is covered with the wine mixture. Simmer over low heat for about 30 minutes or until the meat is tender. Sprinkle with parsley. Salt and pepper to taste. When ready to serve the sauce should be thick and creamy.

Combine salad dressing ingredients, shake well and pour 2 Tablespoons over the lettuce. Mix well, divide and place in bowls. Cut Grapes in half. Divide mandarin oranges, strawberries and grapes. Place on top of the lettuce. (You can omit the strawberries, grapes or mandarin oranges and still have a balanced meal.)

Divide and weigh each meal to assure the meals all weigh the same, within a few tenths of an ounce.

Dinner - 4 Blocks

Steak and Fries for 3   P   C   F

		P	C	F
12 oz.	Bottom Round Steak	80.2	0	12.8
1	Garlic Clove, small	0	0	0
½ t	Pepper	0	0	0
-	Salt to taste	0	0	0
1½ T	Canola Oil	0	0	21.0
-	Fat Free Cooking Spray	0	0	0
4	Red Potatoes (about 24 oz.)	7.7	55.7	0
-	Salt	0	0	0
-	Pepper	0	0	0

Mandarin Orange Salad:

		P	C	F
1 C	Romaine Lettuce	3.0	5.0	0
½ C	Mandarin Oranges, light	1.0	16.0	0
15	Grapes	0	7.5	0
2 C	Strawberries, sliced	2.0	14.0	0
1 T	Sugar	0	9.0	0
2 T	Mandarin Orange Salad Dressing	0	6.0	2.2
		93.9	113.2	36.0
		11.8	12.5	12.0
		3.9	4.1	4.0

Mandarin Orange Salad Dressing:

1 t	Canola Oil
3 T	Mandarin Orange liquid, light
1 t	Red Wine Vinegar
1 t	Cider Vinegar
1 t	Sugar

Fries:

Preheat oven to 500 degrees. Spray 2 large cookie sheets with a fat free cooking spray. Wash potatoes, cut out eyes and slice to ¼" thick. Place potatoes in a bowl and toss with the Canola Oil, salt and pepper. Divide potato slices evenly between pans. Bake about 20 minutes or until tender and lightly browned.

Cut all visible fat from the steak before weighing. Place steak on a plate and rub with salt, pepper and garlic. Heat Grill on medium high. Grill steak about 14 minutes for medium-rare or until desired doneness, turning once.

Remove steak to cutting board and thinly slice steak diagonally across the grain.

Divide and weigh each meal to assure the meals all weigh the same, within a few tenths of an ounce.

Dinner - 4 Blocks

Bottom Round Roast and Vegetables for 3

		P	C	F
12 oz	Bottom Round Roast	79.9	0	24.8
-	Fat Free Cooking Spray	0	0	0
1 T	Butter	0	0	11.0
½ t	Dried Thyme Leaves	0	0	0
½ t	Pepper	0	0	0
1	Bay Leaf	0	0	0
1 C	Carrots, sliced	2.0	23.0	0
6	Potatoes, New Red, small (12 oz.)	4.0	27.8	0
½ C	Onions, chopped	0.9	5.6	0.1
4	Pearl Onions	0.5	6.0	0
½ C	Red Wine	0	0	0
1	Dry Onion Soup Mix	0	16.0	0
2 T	Flour	1.4	11.0	0
¼ C	Mandarin Oranges, light	0.5	8.0	0
10	Grapes	0	5.0	0
1 C	Strawberries, sliced	1.0	7.0	0
2 T	Mandarin Orange Salad Dressing	0	6.0	2.2
		86.2	115.4	38.1
		12.3	12.8	12.7
		4.1	4.2	4.2

Mandarin Orange Salad Dressing: Makes 4 Tablespoons.

1 t	Canola Oil
3 T	Mandarin Orange liquid, light
1 t	Red Wine Vinegar
1 t	Cider Vinegar
1 t	Sugar

Pot Roast:

Preheat oven to 350-degrees. Wipe beef with damp paper towel. Place a piece of heavy foil in a shallow roasting pan. Center roast on foil; rub with thyme, pepper and bay leaf. Surround with potatoes and carrots. Pour the wine over the roast and sprinkle roast and vegetables with the soup mix. Seal foil at the top and sides. Roast in oven for about 1½ hours, or until fork-tender.

Remove roast from oven and transfer to a warm platter. Arrange vegetables around the roast. Strain the pan drippings, pressing any vegetable bits through a sieve into a 2-cup measure. Add wine to make 1¾ C liquid and put mixture into a saucepan. Mix flour with 2T of water until smooth. Stir into drippings in saucepan; bring to a boil, stirring with a wooden spoon. Reduce heat and simmer 3 minutes. Serve gravy over meat and vegetables.

Divide and weigh each meal to assure the meals all weigh the same, within a few tenths of an ounce.

Dinner - 3 Blocks

Moussaka for 6		**P**	**C**	**F**
20 oz.	Hamburger, 93% lean	105.0	0	30.0
1½ T	Olive Oil	0	0	21.0
-	Fat Free Cooking Spray	0	0	0
1	Eggplant (about 16 oz.)	4.7	16.3	0.8
3 C	Zucchini, sliced	6.0	12.0	0
1 med.	Onion	1.8	11.2	0.2
2 T	Parsley	0	0	0
1 t	Salt	0	0	0
1 t	Oregano	0	0	0
4.5 oz.	Mushrooms, drained	1.0	2.0	0
7¼ oz.	Pimiento	2.1	9.5	0.8
6 oz.	Tomato Paste	5.0	25.0	0
6 drops	Tobasco	0	0	0
1 Can	Cheddar Cheese Soup	5.2	13.1	7.8
4 T	Parmesan Cheese, grated, fat free	2.0	6.0	0
2 Cans	Mandarin Oranges, light (11 oz each)	0	76.0	0
6 T	Cool Whip, fat free	0	9.0	0
		132.8	180.1	60.6
		18.9	20.0	20.2
		3.1	3.3	3.3

Slice the eggplant, zucchini and onions and set aside.

Spray a cool skillet with fat free cooking spray add the olive oil. Add the hamburger and onion. Cook until beef is brown, stirring occasionally.

Stir in the sliced eggplant, zucchini and onion. Cook for about 3 minutes then add the next 8 ingredients. Let it cook down until the vegetables are tender.

Divide and weigh each meal to assure the meals all weigh the same, within a few tenths of an ounce.

Serve mandarin oranges and fat free whipped topping for dessert.

Dinner - 4 Blocks

Beef Bourguignon for 4   P   C   F

		P	C	F
16 oz.	Bottom Round, lean	107.5	0	17.2
-	Fat Free Cooking Spray	0	0	0
3 T	Butter	0	0	33.0
2 T	Brandy	0	0	0
6	Pearl Onions	0.6	7.5	0
1 C	Mushrooms, small, whole	0.6	0.9	0.1
2 T	Cornstarch	0	14.0	0
1	Beef Bouillon Cube	0	1.0	0
1 T	Tomato Paste	0.5	2.5	0
½ can	Beef Broth, condensed	3.7	1.2	0
¾ C	Burgundy Wine	0	0	0
½ C	Dry Sherry	0	0	0
½ C	Ruby Port	0	0	0
1	Bay Leaf	0	0	0
-	Chopped Parsley	0	0	0
1½ C	Egg Noodles, dry	8.0	38.0	2.5
1 C	Romaine Lettuce	3.0	5.0	0
4	Peaches, fresh	0	36.0	0
30	Grapes	0	15.0	0
3 C	Strawberries, diced	3.0	21.0	0
1½ T	Sugar	0	18.0	0
2 T	Mandarin Orange Salad Dressing	0	6.0	2.2
		126.9	162.6	55.0
		18.1	18.0	18.3
		4.5	4.5	4.5

    Preheat oven to 350 degrees.

    Cut beef into 1½" cubes. Coat with the cornstarch; (shake off excess cornstarch and reserve). Spray a 3-quart Dutch oven (with a tight-fitting lid) with fat free cooking spray. Add 2 tablespoons of butter, and heat. Add beef, a few at a time, until all the pieces are brown.

    In a small saucepan, heat 2 T brandy just until vapor rises. Ignite; pour over beef. As flame dies, remove beef cubes to another pan and set aside. Melt 1 tablespoon of butter in Dutch oven, add onions, and cook over low heat, covered, until onions brown slightly, stirring occasionally. Then add the mushrooms, cook, stirring about 3 minutes. With slotted spoon, remove onions and mushrooms. Remove Dutch oven from heat. Using a wooden spoon, stir in reserved cornstarch, tomato paste and blend well. Stir in Burgundy, sherry, port and beef broth.

    Bring wine mixture just to a boil, stirring; remove from heat. Add beef, pepper, bay leaf, onions, mushrooms and remaining brandy; mix well. Place a large sheet of waxed paper over top of the Dutch oven; place lid on top of paper. Bake, covered. Stir occasionally, cook 1 hour, or until beef is tender when pierced with a fork. Pour off liquid collected on paper. Sprinkle with parsley. Serve over egg noodles. Have a fruit salad for dessert.

    Divide and weigh each meal to assure the meals all weigh the same, within a few tenths of an ounce.

Dinner -4 Blocks

Beef Liver Smothered in Onions for 3

		P	C	F
12 oz	Beef Liver	67.8	19.8	12.9
½ C	Milk*	0	0	0
2 T	Flour	1.4	11.0	0
-	Fat Free Cooking Spray	0	0	0
2 T	Butter	0	0	22.0
24 oz	Onions, sliced	7.0	43.0	1.0
1 Can	Asparagus	7.0	7.0	0
1 t	Butter	0	0	3.6

Mandarin Orange Salad:

1 C	Romaine Lettuce	3.0	5.0	0
1 C	Strawberries	1.0	7.0	0
30	Grapes	0	15.0	0
1 T	Mandarin Orange Salad Dressing	0	3.0	1.1
		87.2	110.8	39.6
		12.4	12.3	13.2
		4.1	4.1	4.4

Mandarin Orange Salad Dressing:

1 t	Canola Oil
3 T	Mandarin Orange liquid, light
1 t	Red Wine Vinegar
1 t	Cider Vinegar
1 t	Sugar

Place liver in a bowl, pour in ½ C of milk, cover and refrigerate at least one hour or overnight to sweeten the liver and remove any trace of bitterness. Discard the milk when ready to prepare meal.

Spray a cool skillet with fat free cooking spray, add the butter and heat. Slice the onions in rings and fry until they are done to your taste. Peel off the thin membrane that surrounds the liver and cut away any connective tissue. (It shrinks when cooked and will cause liver to warp or curl.)

Dust the liver with flour. Remove the onions and cover to keep warm. Add the liver to the skillet. Fry the liver for 1 ½ to 3 minutes on each side, depending on the thickness (for medium rare) or until it is browned all over. (If liver is cooked too long it becomes tough and bitter tasting so it's better-served medium rare. When properly cooked, liver is juicy, pink inside and as flavorful as a steak.) Transfer liver to 3 warmed plates and top with onions.

Heat asparagus and melt ½ teaspoon of butter over top. Serve with the fruit salad.
*Milk is not added to the PCF count as it is not absorbed.

Divide and weigh each meal to assure the meals all weigh the same, within a few tenths of an ounce.

Dinner - 4 Blocks

	Roast Beef with Vegetables for 6	P	C	F
24 oz.	Beef Top Round	147.8	0	25.4
-	Fat Free Cooking Spray	0	0	0
-	Meat Tenderizer	0	0	0
3 T	Butter	0	0	33.0
-	Salt and Pepper to taste	0	0	0
2	Beef Bouillon Cubes	0	2.0	0
18	Potatoes, Red small chunks (36 oz.)	12.0	84.0	0
2 can	Green Beans	2.0	27.0	0
4.5 oz.	Mushrooms (canned)	6.0	4.0	0
12 slices	Wheat Bread, Pepperidge Farm, light	28.0	88.0	4.0
1½ T	Butter	0	0	16.5

	Mandarin Orange Salad:			
1 C	Romaine Lettuce	3.0	5.0	0
¼ C	Mandarin Oranges, light	0.5	8.0	0
30	Grapes	0	15.0	0
1 T	Mandarin Orange Salad Dressing	0	3.0	1.1
		199.3	236.0	80.0
		28.4	26.2	26.6
		4.7	4.3	4.4

Mandarin Orange Salad Dressing:
1 t	Canola Oil
3 T	Mandarin Orange liquid, light
1 t	Red Wine Vinegar
1 t	Cider Vinegar
1 t	Sugar

Spray a cool skillet with fat free cooking spray; add the butter and heat. Sprinkle the roast with meat tenderizer and, using a fork, stab the tenderizer into meat. Add beef roast to the skillet and brown on both sides. Turn down heat; add the bouillon cubes and some water. Cook slowly until almost tender. (Keep adding water as needed to keep the roast from burning.) Add the mushrooms, potatoes and green beans with it's liquid and continue cooking until beef is tender and the potatoes are done. Adding a small amount of water to keep the roast from getting dry.

Combine salad dressing ingredients, shake well and pour 2 Tablespoons over the lettuce. Mix well, divide and place in bowls. Cut Grapes in half. Divide mandarin oranges and grapes. Place on top of the lettuce.

Divide and weigh beef, and vegetables (within a few 10th of an oz.) to assure the meals are equal.

Chicken Dinner Choices

Dinner - 5 Blocks

Oriental Chicken for 3

		P	C	F
12 oz	Chicken Breasts, skinless, boneless	78.0	0	4.8
2 T	Oriental Sesame Oil	0	0	27.2
5 T	Soy Sauce	5.0	5.0	0
2 T	Brown Sugar	0	24.0	0
2 T	Water	0	0	0
1	Garlic Clove, chopped	0	0	0
1 t	Ground Ginger	0	0	0
1 oz	Cashews, (14 large or 26 small)	5.0	8.0	13.0
1 C	Snow Peas	4.0	12.0	0
¼ C	White Rice raw (1 cup cooked)	4.0	38.0	0
2 C	Romaine Lettuce, or any leafy lettuce	6.0	10.0	0
¼ C	Mandarin Oranges, light	0.5	8.0	0
20	Grapes	0	10.0	0
1½ C	Strawberries	1.5	14.0	0
1 t	Sugar	0	4.0	0
2 T	Mandarin Orange Salad Dressing	0	6.0	2.2
		108.0	139.0	47.2
		15.4	15.4	15.7
		5.1	5.1	5.2

Mandarin Orange Salad Dressing: Makes 4 Tablespoons.

1 t	Canola Oil
3 T	Mandarin Orange liquid, light
1 t	Red Wine Vinegar
1 t	Cider Vinegar
1 t	Sugar

Put the Sesame Oil in a skillet and brown chicken on both sides, over medium heat. Combine brown sugar, soy sauce, water, garlic and ginger. Pour over chicken, cover and cook about 30 minutes, or until chicken is no longer pink.

Meanwhile, cook the rice, following the package directions, but don't add any butter. When rice is almost done steam the snow peas.

When rice is done, divide and put on 3 plates then put one piece of chicken on each plate. Divide the sauce and pour over chicken. Sprinkle with cashews and serve with the snow peas and rice.

Divide and weigh each meal to assure the meals all weigh the same, within a few tenths of an ounce.

Dinner 4- Blocks

Cranberry Chicken for 3

		P	C	F
12 oz	Chicken Breasts, skinless, boneless	78.0	0	4.8
-	Fat Free Cooking Spray	0	0	0
1 T	Butter	0	0	11.0
1 C	Water	0	0	0
-	Salt and Pepper to taste	0	0	0
½ C	Cranberries, fresh or frozen	0.2	4.0	0.1
¼ C	Brown Sugar, unpacked	0	70.5	0
½ T	Red Wine Vinegar	0	0	0
-	Nutmeg, dash	0	0	0
1 C	Cauliflower	2.0	5.0	0
1 C	Brussels Sprouts	6.0	20.0	1.0
½ C	Carrots	1.0	11.5	0
2 T	Butter	0	0	22.0
		87.2	111.0	38.9
		12.4	12.3	12.9
		4.1	4.1	4.3

Spray a cool skillet with fat free cooking spray; add the butter and heat.

Combine the flour, salt and pepper and coat the chicken. Reserve remaining flour. Place chicken breasts in the skillet and brown all over. Remove the chicken and set aside.

In the same skillet, combine cranberries, brown sugar, red wine vinegar water and nutmeg. Cover and simmer for about 5 minutes. Return the chicken to the skillet, cover and simmer for 20 to 25 minutes, or until the chicken is no longer pink.

Meanwhile, prepare the vegetables and steam until crisp tender. Put the vegetables in a bowl and melt the 2 T of butter over them. Serve.

Divide and weigh each meal to assure the meals all weigh the same, within a few tenths of an ounce.

Dinner - 4 Blocks

Honey Orange Chicken Stir-Fry for 3

		P	C	F
9 oz.	Chicken Breasts, skinless, boneless	58.5	0	3.6
-	Fat Free Cooking Spray	0	0	0
1 T	Canola Oil	0	0	14.0
½ t	Orange Peel, grated	0	0	0
1 T	Cornstarch	0	7.0	0
½ T	Honey	0	8.0	0
3 oz.	Orange Juice	0.7	9.7	0
¼ C	White Rice, raw (1 Cup cooked)	4.0	38.0	0
26	Cashews, large	5.0	8.0	13.0
1 can	Asparagus	7.0	7.0	0
½ T	Butter	0	0	5.5
2 C	Romaine Lettuce	6.0	10.0	0
1 C	Strawberries, sliced	1.0	7.0	0
15	Grapes	0	7.5	0
1 T	Mandarin Orange Salad Dressing	0	3.0	1.1
		82.2	105.2	37.2
		11.7	11.6	12.4
		3.9	3.8	4.1

Mandarin Orange Salad Dressing: Makes 4 Tablespoons.

1 t	Canola Oil
3 T	Mandarin Orange liquid, light
1 t	Red Wine Vinegar
1 t	Cider Vinegar
1 t	Sugar

Prepare rice according to the directions on the package but omit the butter.

Cut chicken into thin slices. Spray a cool wok with fat free cooking spray; add the oil and heat. Add chicken to the wok and fry until chicken is no longer pink and the juices run clear. In a small bowl, combine orange juice, honey, cornstarch, and orange peel. Blend the mixture well and add to wok.

Cook, stirring until mixture thickens. Divide chicken, mixture, and rice. Put on a plate. Divide cashews and put on top just before serving. Heat the asparagus, drain liquid and melt 1 T of butter over top.

Combine salad dressing ingredients, shake well and pour 1 Tablespoon over the lettuce. Mix well, divide and place in bowls. Cut the grapes in half. Divide mandarin oranges, grapes and strawberries. Place on top of the lettuce.

Divide and weigh each meal to assure the meals all weigh the same, within a few tenths of an ounce.

Dinner - 4 Blocks

Chicken Breasts with Sour Cherry Sauce for 3

		P	C	F
12 oz.	Chicken Breasts (3 breasts, 4 oz. each)	78.0	0	4.8
-	Fat Free Cooking Spray	0	0	0
2 T	Butter	0	0	22.0
½ C	White Wine	0	0	0
5.5 oz.	Sour Cherries in water, (¾ C)	3.0	18.0	0
¼ C	Sugar	0	36.0	0
1½ T	Cornstarch	0	10.5	0
½ C	Cherry liquid (¼ C)	0	4.0	0
-	Salt, to taste	0	0	0
11 oz.	Corn (canned)	8.0	40.0	2.0
1 Can	Green Beans	3.5	10.5	0
1 T	Butter	0	0	11.0
Fruit Salad:				
¼ C	Mandarin Oranges, light	0.5	8.0	0
1 C	Strawberries	1.0	7.0	0
		94.0	134.0	39.8
		13.4	14.8	13.2
		4.4	4.9	4.4

Chicken:

Spray a cool skillet with fat free cooking spray. Add 2 T butter and heat. Add the chicken to the hot skillet and brown on both sides. Sprinkle chicken with about ¼ t salt. Add white wine and simmer chicken until chicken is no longer pink and the juice runs clear. (About 10 minutes)

Meanwhile, in a 2-qt. saucepan, combine cornstarch, cherry liquid and sugar. Heat to a boil, stirring constantly, until sauce thickens. Stir in salt to taste (about ¼ t) and the pitted cherries. Cook until cherries are heated through.

When chicken is done, using a slotted spoon, transfer to a serving platter. (Cover to keep warm) Add the cherries and cornstarch mixture to the skillet.

Divide the cherries and sauce equally and spoon over the chicken on the platter. Serve with heated vegetables and fruit salad.

Divide and weigh each meal to assure the meals all weigh the same, within a few tenths of an ounce.

You can omit the fruit salad and still have a balanced meal.

Dinner - 4 Blocks

Chicken Thighs with Sour Cherry Sauce for 3		P	C	F
12 oz.	Chicken Thighs, skinless, boneless	67.2	0	13.2
-	Fat Free Cooking Spray	0	0	0
1½ T	Butter	0	0	16.5
½ C	White Wine	0	0	0
5.5 oz.	Sour Cherries in water, (¾ C)	3.0	18.0	0
¼ C	Sugar	0	36.0	0
1½ T	Cornstarch	0	10.5	0
¼ C	Cherry liquid	0	4.0	0
¼ C	Water	0	0	0
-	Salt, to taste	0	0	0
11 oz.	Corn (canned)	8.0	40.0	2.0
1 can	Green Beans	3.5	10.5	0
2 t	Butter	0	0	7.2
Fruit Salad:				
1 C	Strawberries	1.0	7.0	0
		82.7	126.0	38.9
		11.8	14.0	12.9
		3.9	4.6	4.3

Chicken:

Spray a cool skillet with fat free cooking spray. Add 1½ T butter and heat. Add the chicken to the hot skillet and brown on both sides. Sprinkle chicken with about ¼ t salt. Add white wine and simmer chicken until chicken is no longer pink and the juice runs clear. (About 10 minutes)

Meanwhile, in a 2-qt. saucepan, combine cornstarch, cherry liquid, water and sugar.

When chicken is done, using a slotted spoon, transfer to a serving platter. (Cover to keep warm) Add the cornstarch mixture to the skillet. Heat to a boil, stirring constantly, until sauce thickens. Stir in salt to taste (about ¼ t) and the pitted cherries. Cook until cherries are heated through.

Divide the cherries and sauce equally and spoon over the chicken on the platter. Serve with heated vegetables and fruit salad.

Divide and weigh each meal to assure the meals all weigh the same, within a few tenths of an ounce.

You can omit the fruit salad and still have a balanced meal.

Dinner - 4 Blocks

Chicken Cutlet Parmesan in Tomato Sauce for 3

		P	C	F
9 oz.	Chicken Breasts, skinless, boneless	58.5	0	3.6
-	Fat Free Cooking Spray	0	0	0
1 ½ T	Olive Oil	0	0	21.0
1 T	Italian Seasoned Bread Crumbs	1.0	4.5	0.4
1 T	Parmesan Cheese, fat free	1.5	4.5	0
1 slice	Mozzarella Cheese (1.5 oz.)	12.0	0	8.0
2 oz	Angel Hair Spaghetti	7.0	40.0	1.0
1 C	Romaine Lettuce	3.0	5.0	0
2 C	Strawberries, sliced	2.0	14.0	1.2
30	Grapes	0	15.0	0
1 T	Mandarin Orange Salad Dressing	0	3.0	1.1

Tomato Sauce:

		P	C	F
1 C	Onion, diced	1.8	11.2	0.2
1	Garlic Clove, minced	0	0	0
15 oz	Diced Tomatoes, Italian Style Herbs	3.0	12.0	0
½ C	Tomato Sauce	1.0	4.0	0
½ t	Sugar	0	2.0	0
2 t	Oregano, dried	0	0	0
		90.8	115.2	36.5
		12.9	12.8	12.1
		4.3	4.2	4.0

Mandarin Orange Salad Dressing: Makes 4 Tablespoons.

1 t	Canola Oil
3 T	Mandarin Orange liquid, light
1 t	Red Wine Vinegar
1 t	Cider Vinegar
1 t	Sugar

Tomato Sauce:

    Place all tomato sauce ingredients in a saucepan and bring to a boil. Reduce heat to low and simmer about 30 minutes, or until the sauce is thick.

    Spray cool skillet with a fat free cooking spray; add the olive oil and heat. Coat the chicken with the breadcrumbs. (Remove any fat and bone before weighing.) Place the breaded chicken into the heated skillet and brown on all sides until the chicken is no longer pink and the juices run clear. Cut the mozzarella cheese into 3 equal portions and place on top of each piece of chicken. Cover and heat until the cheese has melted.

    Cook the spaghetti. Divide and place on a plate. Place a piece of chicken on top; add 1/3 of the sauce. Divide the Parmesan cheese, sprinkle over the sauce and serve.

    Combine salad dressing ingredients, shake well and pour 1 Tablespoon over the lettuce. Mix well, divide and place in bowls. Divide mandarin oranges and place on top of the lettuce.

    Divide and weigh each meal to assure the meals all weigh the same, within a few tenths of an ounce.

Dinner - 4 Blocks

Chicken and Artichokes for 3

		P	C	F
9 oz.	Chicken Breasts, skinless, boneless	58.5	0	3.6
-	Fat Free Cooking Spray	0	0	0
1 T	Butter	0	0	11.0
½ t	Salt	0	0	0
¼ t	Pepper	0	0	0
½ t	Oregano, dried	0	0	0
1 C	Mushrooms, fresh, sliced	2.0	4.0	0
12 oz.	Artichoke Hearts, canned	11.7	34.2	0.6
4 slices	Lemon, thin	0	2.0	0
1 T	Flour	0.7	5.5	0
½ C	White Wine	0	0	0
3 oz.	Egg Noodles, 2 C dry	8.0	38.0	2.4
1 can	Asparagus	7.0	7.0	0
1 T	Butter	0	0	11.0
1 C	Romaine Lettuce	3.0	5.0	0
1 C	Strawberries, sliced	1.0	7.0	0
6	Grapes	0	2.5	0
1 T	Mandarin Orange Salad Dressing	0	3.0	1.1
1 T	Almond, slivered	3.0	3.0	8.0
		94.9	111.2	37.1
		13.5	12.3	12.3
		4.5	4.1	4.1

Mandarin Orange Salad Dressing: Makes 4 Tablespoons.
- 1 t   Canola Oil
- 3 T   Mandarin Orange liquid, light
- 1 t   Red Wine Vinegar
- 1 t   Cider Vinegar
- 1 t   Sugar

Combine salad dressing ingredients, shake well and pour 1 Tablespoon over the lettuce. Mix well, divide and place in bowls. Cut grapes in half. Divide strawberries, grapes and mandarin oranges, place on top of lettuce. Divide the almonds and sprinkle on top of salad.

Cook the egg noodles according to the directions on the package

Spray a cool skillet with fat free cooking spray and heat. Season chicken with the salt and pepper and oregano. Brown about 3 minutes each side. Remove from skillet and keep warm. In the same skillet, add 1 Tablespoon of butter and the mushrooms and cook until tender, about 3 minutes. Add artichoke hearts and cook about 1 minute, until heated through. Mix the wine, lemon juice and flour and add to the skillet. Bring to a boil, stirring continuously until mixture thickens, about 5 minutes. Return the chicken to the skillet and heat. Divide egg noodles and place on each plate. Place chicken on the noodles and pour the sauce over the chicken. Heat the asparagus, drain liquid and melt 1 Tablespoon of butter over the top.

Divide and weigh each meal to assure the meals all weigh the same, within a few tenths of an ounce.

Dinner - 4 Blocks

Manhattan Chicken for 3

		P	C	F
9 oz.	Chicken Breasts, skinless, boneless	58.5	0	3.6
1 slice	Wheat Bread, Pepperidge Farm, light	2.0	7.0	0
-	Fat Free Cooking Spray	0	0	0
1 T	Canola Oil	0	0	14.0
1 T	Butter	0	0	11.0
1	Egg White	4.0	0	0
1 C	Mushrooms, fresh, sliced	2.0	4.0	0
1	Garlic Clove	0	0	0
10 oz.	Frozen Spinach	6.9	9.3	0.5
½ t	Nutmeg	0	0	0
¼ C	White Wine	0	0	0
1 oz.	Provolone Cheese	7.0	1.0	5.0
1½ C	White Rice, cooked	6.0	57.0	0
1 can	Green Beans	3.0	6.0	0
1 C	Romaine Lettuce	3.0	5.0	0
1 C	Strawberries, sliced	1.0	7.0	0
10	Grapes	0	5.0	0
1 T	Mandarin Orange Salad Dressing	0	3.0	1.1
		93.4	104.3	35.2
		13.3	11.5	11.7
		4.4	3.8	3.9

Mandarin Orange Salad Dressing: Makes 4 Tablespoons.

1 t	Canola Oil
3 T	Mandarin Orange liquid, light
1 t	Red Wine Vinegar
1 t	Cider Vinegar
1 t	Sugar

   Combine salad dressing ingredients, shake well and pour 1 Tablespoon over the lettuce. Mix well, divide and place in bowls. Cut grapes in half. Divide strawberries and grapes and place on top of lettuce.

   Spray a cool skillet with fat free cooking spray, and then add oil and butter. Heat. Toast the bread and crumble as fine as you can. Coat the chicken with egg and then the breadcrumbs. Place chicken in skillet and brown all over. Add next 5 ingredients. Cook until chicken is no longer pink and the juices run clear. Place cheese on top of chicken breasts, cover and heat until cheese melts. Serve over rice.

   Divide and weigh each meal to assure the meals all weigh the same, within a few tenths of an ounce.

Dinner - 4 Blocks

Chicken with Orange Peel Szechwan Style for 3		P	C	F
12 oz.	Chicken Breasts, skinless, boneless	78.0	0	4.8
-	Fat Free Cooking Spray	0	0	0
1 T	Olive Oil	0	0	14.0
3 T	Orange Peel	0.3	3.9	0.1
1 T	Soy Sauce	1.0	1.0	0
1 T	Dry Sherry	0	0	0
¼ C	Green Onions, (cut in 2" pieces)	0.5	1.2	0
¼ t	Crushed Red Pepper	0	0	0
1 t	Ginger Root, minced	0	0	0
1 T	Cornstarch	0	7.0	0
-	Salt to taste	0	0	0
½ t	Sugar	0	2.0	0
½ C	Orange Juice	0.8	13.0	0
1½ C	White Rice, cooked	6.0	57.0	0
½ C	Carrots, raw	1.0	11.5	0
½ C	Snow Peas, raw	2.0	6.0	0
1 C	Brussels Sprouts	6.0	20.0	1.0
2 T	Butter	0	0	22.0
		95.6	122.6	41.9
		13.6	13.6	13.9
		4.5	4.5	4.6

With potato peeler, cut peel from orange into 1½" pieces, being careful not to cut into the white. Heat the oven to 200 degrees. Spread orange peel pieces on a cookie sheet, put in the oven, and let them dry slightly for about 30 minutes.

Cut chicken into about 1½" strips. In a medium bowl, mix chicken strips, soy sauce, green onions, sherry, red pepper and ginger. In a small bowl, mix cornstarch, salt orange juice and sugar. Cover both bowls and refrigerate until ready to stir-fry.

Spray a cool wok with fat free cooking spray, add the oil and quickly stir-fry the slightly dried orange peel strips. Stir frequently, until peels are crisp and the edges are slightly brown. (About 2 minutes) Remove from the wok and cool on a paper towel. Add the chicken mixture to the oil in the skillet, over high heat; stir-fry the chicken until no longer pink. (About 4 minutes) Stir orange juice mixture and add to the chicken. Stir-fry until mixture is slightly thickened. Spoon over rice; divide the orange peel and place on top of the chicken mixture and serve. Steam vegetables on separate sides of the steamer. Divide each vegetable by 3 and place on plates. Divide the butter by 3 and melt over the vegetables.

Divide and weigh each meal to assure the meals all weigh the same, within a few tenths of an ounce.

Dinner - 4 Blocks

Chicken with Peach Sauté for 3   P   C   F

		P	C	F
12 oz.	Chicken Breasts, skinless, boneless	78.0	0	4.8
-	Fat Free Cooking Spray	0	0	0
2½ T	Canola Oil	0	0	35.0
¼ C	Green Pepper, wedges	0.2	2.8	0
¼ C	Onions, wedged	0.5	2.8	0
2 oz.	Orange Juice	0.4	6.5	0
2 T	Sugar	0	24.0	0
2 t	Cornstarch	0	4.6	0
½ t	Ginger	0	0	0
¼ t	Paprika	0	0	0
-	Pepper to taste	0	0	0
1 C	Peaches, sliced thin	1.2	16.2	0
1½ C	White Rice, cooked	6.0	57.0	0
1 Can	Green Beans	3.5	10.5	0
		90.1	124.4	39.8
		12.8	13.8	13.2
		4.2	4.6	4.4

Prepare rice as directed on package but omit the butter.

In a small bowl, combine orange juice, sugar, cornstarch, ginger, paprika and pepper to taste. Blend well and set aside. Spray a cool wok with fat free cooking spray. Heat oil in wok on medium high heat. Add chicken; cook 4 to 6 minutes or until lightly brown, stirring continuously. Add peppers and onions.

Cook and stir 4 to 5 minutes more, until chicken is no longer pink and the vegetables are crisp-tender.

Stir the orange juice mixture and pour over the chicken. Add the peaches and cook another 2 or 3 minutes, until the sauce is thick and bubbly. Serve over rice. Heat green beans.

Divide and weigh each meal to assure the meals all weigh the same, within a few tenths of an ounce.

Dinner - 4 Blocks

Hawaiian Chicken for 3

		P	C	F
12 oz.	Chicken Breasts (4 oz. each)	78.0	0	4.8
-	Fat Free Cooking Spray	0	0	0
2½ T	Olive Oil	0	0	34.0
3 T	Sugar	0	36.0	0
1 T	Cider Vinegar	0	0	0
1 T	Cornstarch	0	7.0	0
1 t	Soy Sauce	0.5	0.5	0
¼ t	Ginger Root	0	0	0
1	Chicken Bouillon Cube	0	1.0	0
3	Green Pepper Rings, ¼" thick	0.2	2.8	0
3	Pineapple Rings, in juice	0	21.0	0
¼ C	White Rice, raw (1 Cup when cooked)	4.0	38.0	0
1 can	Green Beans	3.5	10.5	0
		86.2	116.8	38.8
		12.3	12.9	12.9
		4.1	4.3	4.3

Heat oven to 350 degrees

Prepare rice as directed on package but omit the butter.

Chicken:
Spray a cool skillet with fat free cooking spray. Add the olive oil and heat. Add the chicken to the hot skillet and brown on both sides. Transfer the chicken to an 8" x 8" x 2" baking dish and set aside.

Sauce:
Drain the pineapple, reserving the juice. Transfer the juice to a 1 C measuring cup. Add enough water to make 1 Cup of liquid. In a medium saucepan, using a wire whisk, stir together the juice mixture, sugar, vinegar, cornstarch, soy sauce, ginger and bouillon cube. Bring to a boil over medium heat. Reduce the heat and gently boil for about 4 minutes, stirring often, until it thickens.

Pour half the sauce over the chicken. Arrange the pineapple slices and pepper rings on top. Pour on the rest of the sauce mixture. Bake for 30 to 40 minutes or until the chicken is tender and no linger pink. Serve over rice. Heat the green beans.

Divide and weigh each meal to assure the meals all weigh the same, within a few tenths of an ounce.

Dinner - 4 Blocks

Chicken Cacciatore for 3		P	C	F
12 oz.	Chicken Breasts, skinless, boneless	77.8	0	4.8
-	Fat Free Cooking Spray	0	0	0
-	Salt and Pepper to taste	0	0	0
1 t	Butter	0	0	3.6
2 T	Olive Oil	0	0	28.0
½ C	Onions, diced	0.9	5.6	0
1 C	Green Pepper, diced	0.8	11.2	0.2
½ t	Garlic Powder	0	0	0
½ C	Red Wine	0	0	0
½ t	Oregano	0	0	0
½ t	Basil	0	0	0
1 t	Parsley	0	0	0
14.5 oz.	Italian Tomatoes, canned	3.5	17.5	0
1 can	Green Beans	1.0	10.5	0
1 t	Butter	0	0	3.6
1½ C	White Rice, cooked	6.0	57.0	0

Mandarin Orange Salad:

		P	C	F
2 C	Romaine Lettuce	6.0	10.0	0
6	Grapes	0	2.5	0
1 C	Strawberries, sliced	1.0	7.0	0
1 T	Mandarin Orange Salad Dressing	0	3.0	1.1
	97.0	124.3	37.7
	13.8	13.8	12.5
	4.6	4.6	4.1

Mandarin Orange Salad Dressing: Makes 4 Tablespoons.
1 t Canola Oil
3 T Mandarin Orange liquid, light
1 t Red Wine Vinegar
1 t Cider Vinegar
1 t Sugar

    Prepare rice as directed on package but omit the butter.
    Lightly spray cool skillet with fat free cooking spray; add the oil and butter and heat. Sprinkle chicken with salt and pepper. Fry about 4 minutes or until chicken is lightly browned on both sides. Add onions, green pepper, and garlic powder to the skillet. Stir in wine, tomatoes, oregano, basil and parsley. Bring to a boil; reduce heat to medium low. Cover and simmer for about 30 minutes or until chicken is tender and no longer pink. Serve over rice. Heat green beans and divide into 3 portions.

    Combine salad dressing ingredients, shake well and pour 1 Tablespoon over the lettuce, mix well, divide and place in bowls. Divide grapes and strawberries, place on top of lettuce.
    (You can omit the strawberries and/or grapes and still be balanced.)

    Divide and weigh each meal to assure the meals all weigh the same, within a few tenths of an ounce.

Dinner - 4 Blocks

Chicken a la Marengo for 3

		P	C	F
12 oz.	Chicken Breasts, skinless, boneless	78.0	0	4.8
-	Fat Free Cooking Spray	0	0	0
1½ T	Olive Oil	0	0	21.0
14 oz.	Stewed Tomato, recipe style	3.5	24.5	0
1 C	Onions, chopped	1.8	11.2	0.2
¼ t	Garlic Powder	0	0	0
1 t	Parsley	0	0	0
¼ t	Thyme	0	0	0
¼ t	Rosemary	0	0	0
¼ C	White Wine	0	0	0
1	Bay Leaf	0	0	0
-	Salt and Pepper to taste	0	0	0
1½ C	White Rice, cooked	6.0	57.0	0
1 can	Asparagus	7.0	7.0	0
1½ T	Butter	0	0	16.5
10	Grapes	0	5.0	0
¼ C	Mandarin Oranges, light	0.5	8.0	0
1 C	Strawberries, sliced	1.0	7.0	0
		97.8	19.7	42.5
		13.9	13.3	14.1
		4.6	4.4	4.7

Prepare rice as directed on package but omit the butter.

Lightly spray a cool skillet with fat free cooking spray. Add the oil.

Over medium heat, add the chicken breasts and brown lightly all over. Remove the chicken. Add onion and garlic. Stir until onions are tender.

Return chicken to the skillet. Sprinkle with thyme, parsley and rosemary. Add the stewed tomatoes and juice, wine and bay leaf. Bring to a boil. Reduce heat, cover and simmer for about 20 minutes or until chicken is tender and no longer pink. Serve over rice.

Heat the asparagus. Divide the asparagus and butter by three and place on individual plates. Divide fruit and put into individual bowls.

Divide and weigh each meal to assure the meals all weigh the same, within a few tenths of an ounce.

Dinner - 4 Blocks

Garlic Chicken with Ham Salad for 3   P   C   F

		P	C	F
12 oz.	Chicken Breasts, skinless, boneless	78.0	0	4.8
3	Garlic Cloves, peeled	0.3	1.4	0
-	Fat Free Cooking Spray	0	0	0
½ T	Olive Oil	0	0	7.7
1 T	White Wine Vinegar	0	0.6	0
¼ C	Chicken Broth	0.2	0.2	0.3
1½ T	Butter	0	0	16.5
½ T	Fresh Tarragon, chopped	0	0	0
¾ C	Carrots, raw	1.5	17.2	0
1 C	Cauliflower, raw	2.0	5.0	0
½ C	Snow Peas, raw	2.0	6.0	0
1 T	Butter	0	0	11.0

Ham Salad:

		P	C	F
2 C	Romaine Lettuce	6.0	10.0	0
1 slice	Honey Ham, 96% lean	5.0	0	1.0
1	Tomato, medium, chopped	1.0	6.0	0
2 T	Green Onion, diced	0.3	0.6	0
6 T	Thousand Island Salad Dressing, fat free	0	12.0	0

Dessert:

		P	C	F
3 C	Strawberries, chopped	3.0	21.0	0
2 t	Sugar	0	8.0	0
1½ C	Cool Whip, fat free	0	36.0	0
		99.3	124.0	41.3
		14.1	13.7	13.47
		4.7	4.5	4.5

Spray a cool skillet with fat free cooking spray; add the olive oil and butter. Brown chicken on all sides. Add the garlic cloves, white wine vinegar, chicken broth and tarragon. Cook over low heat until the chicken is no longer pink and the juices run clear.

Place torn lettuce in 3 bowls. Slice ham and vegetables, divide each by 3, and place on top of the lettuce. Pour 2 Tablespoons of salad dressing over each salad and stir. (You can use any fat free dressing as long as it doesn't raise the carbohydrate block to 5.0.)

Strawberries and cool whip for dessert. (You can substitute 1 Cup of canned sliced Peaches, light, or 2 fresh peaches and still be balanced. Or try another substitution.)

Divide and weigh each meal to assure the meals all weigh the same, within a few tenths of an ounce.

Dinner - 4 Blocks

Garlic Chicken with Angel Food Cake for 3		P	C	F
12 oz.	Chicken Breasts, skinless, boneless	78.0	0	4.8
3	Garlic Cloves, peeled	0.3	1.4	0
-	Fat Free Cooking Spray	0	0	0
½ T	Olive Oil	0	0	7.7
1 T	White Wine Vinegar	0	0.6	0
¼ C	Chicken Broth	0.2	0.2	0.3
1½ T	Butter	0	0	16.5
½ T	Fresh Tarragon, chopped	0	0	0
1 C	Cauliflower, raw	2.0	5.0	0
½ C	Snow Peas, raw	2.0	6.0	0
1 T	Butter	0	0	11.0
Dessert:				
3 slices	1/12th Angel Food Cake	9.0	90.0	0
1½ C	Strawberries, sliced	1.5	10.5	0
6 T	Cool Whip, fat free	0	9.0	0
		93.0	122.7	40.3
		13.2	13.6	13.4
		4.4	4.5	4.4

Bake an Angel Food Cake mix. Divide into 12 equal pieces. The extra pieces can be frozen, or try one of the other recipes that serve Angel Food Cake, strawberries and/or fat free Cool Whip for dessert.

Spray a cool skillet with fat free cooking spray; add the olive oil and butter. Brown chicken on all sides. Add the garlic cloves, white wine vinegar, chicken broth and tarragon. Cook over low heat until the chicken is no longer pink and the juices run clear.

Steam Vegetables, remove from steamer, melt 1 Tablespoon of butter over them, and stir well. Divide into 3 portions. (You don't have to worry if the individual vegetables are divided equally as they have about the same PCF's.)

Angel food cake with strawberries and cool whip for dessert.

(You can substitute 1 Cup of canned sliced Peaches, light, or 2 fresh peaches, or ½ C mandarin oranges, for the strawberries, and still be balanced. Or try another substitution.)

Divide and weigh each meal to assure the meals all weigh the same, within a few tenths of an ounce.

Dinner - 5 Blocks

Chicken Drumsticks with Salad for 3

		P	C	F
6	Chicken Legs, skinless (About 15 oz.)	87.0	0	15.0
2 T	White Flour	1.5	11.0	0
1½ T	Butter	0	0	16.5
½ C	Carrots, raw	1.0	11.5	0
1 C	Cauliflower, raw	2.0	5.0	0
½ C	Snow Peas, raw	2.0	6.0	0
1 C	Brussels Sprouts	6.0	20.0	1.0
1½ T	Butter	0	0	16.5

Mandarin Orange Salad:

		P	C	F
2 C	Romaine Lettuce	6.0	10.0	0
¼ C	Mandarin Oranges, light	0.5	8.0	0
10	Grapes	0	5.0	0
1 T	Mandarin Orange Salad Dressing	0	6.0	1.1

Dessert:

		P	C	F
3 C	Strawberries, sliced	3.0	21.0	0
1 C	Cool Whip, fat free	0	24.0	0
		109.0	127.5	50.1
		15.5	14.1	16.7
		5.1	4.7	5.5

Mandarin Orange Salad Dressing: Makes 4 Tablespoons.

1 t	Canola Oil
3 T	Mandarin Orange liquid, light
1 t	Red Wine Vinegar
1 t	Cider Vinegar
1 t	Sugar

Boil chicken legs until tender, remove the skin then coat with flour. Spray cool skillet with the non-stick spray; add 1½ T butter and fry chicken legs until brown. (The chicken will weigh about 15 ounces after bone is removed.)

Steam vegetables, and melt 1½ Tablespoons of butter on top. Serve with salad. Serve strawberries and cool whip for dessert.

Combine salad dressing ingredients, shake well and pour 2 Tablespoons over the lettuce, mix well, divide and place in bowls. Cut grapes in half. Divide mandarin oranges and grapes and place on top of lettuce.

(1 Cup of canned Peaches, light, or 2 fresh peaches can be substituted for the strawberries and cool whip and still be balanced. Or try another substitution.)

Divide and weigh each meal to assure the meals all weigh the same, within a few tenths of an ounce.

Dinner - 5 Blocks

Chicken Drumsticks with Angel Food Cake for 3		P	C	F
6	Chicken Legs, skinless (About 15 oz.)	87.0	0	15.0
2 T	White Flour	1.5	11.0	0
-	Fat Free Cooking Spray	0	0	0
2 T	Butter	0	0	22.0
1 can	Asparagus	7.0	7.0	0
1 C	Cauliflower, raw	2.0	5.0	0
½ C	Snow Peas, raw	2.0	6.0	0
1 T	Butter	0	0	11.0
Dessert:				
3 slices	1/12th Angel Food Cake	9.0	90.0	0
1½ C	Strawberries, sliced	1.5	10.5	0
15 T	Cool Whip, Fat Free	0	15.0	0
		110.0	144.5	48.0
		15.7	16.0	16.0
		5.2	5.3	5.3

Bake an Angel Food Cake mix. Divide into 12 equal pieces. The extra pieces can be frozen, or try one of the other recipes that serve Angel Food Cake, strawberries and/or fat free Cool Whip for dessert.

Boil chicken legs until tender, remove skin then coat with flour. Spray cool skillet with the fat free cooking spray, add 2 Tablespoon of butter, add chicken and fry until brown. (The chicken will weigh about 15 ounces after bone is removed.)

Steam vegetables, and melt 1 Tablespoon of butter on top.

Serve Angel food cake and strawberries for dessert.

(1 Cup of canned Peaches, light, or 2 fresh peaches, can be substituted for the strawberries and still be balanced. Or try another substitution.)

Divide and weigh each meal to assure the meals all weigh the same, within a few tenths of an ounce.

Dinner - 4 Blocks

Chicken & Stuffing Bake for 3		P	C	F
12 oz.	Chicken Breasts, skinless, boneless	78.0	0	4.8
-	Fat Free Cooking Spray	0	0	0
2 C	Stove Top Chicken Stuffing Mix	12.0	76.0	4.0
2 T	Butter	0	0	22.0
½ can	Cream of Chicken Soup	3.2	7.2	6.4
¼ C	Milk 2%	2.0	3.0	1.2
½ t	Parsley, dried	0	0	0
1 can	Green Beans	1.0	13.5	0

Mandarin Orange Salad:				
1 C	Romaine Lettuce	3.0	5.0	0
¼ C	Mandarin Oranges, light	0.5	8.0	0
1 C	Strawberries, sliced	1.0	7.0	0
1 T	Mandarin Orange Salad Dressing	0	3.0	1.1
		100.7	122.7	39.5
		14.3	13.6	13.1
		4.7	4.5	4.3

Mandarin Orange Salad Dressing: Makes 4 Tablespoons.

1 t	Canola Oil
3 T	Mandarin Orange liquid, light
1 t	Red Wine Vinegar
1 t	Cider Vinegar
1 t	Sugar

Pre-heat the oven to 400 degrees. Spray a cool skillet with fat free cooking spray and brown the chicken. Make the stuffing according to the directions on the box. Spoon 2 Cups of the stuffing mixture down the center of a 3-qt. casserole dish. Arrange chicken breasts on both sides of stuffing. Sprinkle chicken with paprika, salt and pepper. Mix soup, milk and parsley. Pour over chicken. Bake at 400 degrees for 30 minutes, or until chicken is no longer pink and juice runs clear. Serve with Green beans and salad.

Combine salad dressing ingredients, shake well and pour 1 Tablespoon over the lettuce, mix well, divide and place in bowls. Divide mandarin oranges and strawberries, place on top of lettuce.

(You can omit the strawberries and substitute 10 grapes and still have a balanced meal.)

Divide and weigh each meal to assure the meals all weigh the same, within a few tenths of an ounce.

Dinner - 4 Blocks

Teriyaki Chicken with Cole Slaw for 3		P	C	F
12 oz.	Chicken Breasts, skinless, boneless	78.0	0	4.8
3 T	Teriyaki Marinade	3.0	9.0	0
1 C	White Rice, cooked	4.0	38.0	0
1 can	Green Beans	1.5	7.0	0
11 oz.	Corn (canned)	8.0	40.0	2.0
1 T	Butter	0	0	11.0
Cole Slaw:				
2 C	Cabbage, shredded	2.0	8.0	0
3 T	Miracle Whip, regular	0	4.0	21.0
3 T	Miracle Whip, fat free	0	6.0	0
1 T	Vinegar	0	0.3	0
2 t	Sugar	0	8.0	0
		96.5	120.3	38.8
		13.7	13.3	12.9
		4.5	4.4	4.3

Teriyaki Marinade:
¼ C	Light Brown Sugar, packed
¼ C	Soy Sauce
2 T	Lemon Juice
1 T	Canola Oil
¼ t	Ground Ginger
1	Garlic Clove, minced

Makes about 1 cup of marinade. Marinate the chicken in all of it. You will actually use only about 3 tablespoons. Discard leftover marinade.

Prepare rice as directed on package but omit the butter.
Cut chicken in 2-inch squares. Prepare marinade. Place chicken breasts in a large resealable bag. Pour the marinade over chicken and seal the bag. Turn to make sure the chicken is coated all over. Refrigerate for 3 to 6 hours, turning bag occasionally.

Mix miracle whip, vinegar and sugar. Shred cabbage, pour mixture over cabbage and chill.
When ready to cook chicken, heat grill. Place chicken 4" above the heat for 4 to 5 minutes. Turn chicken over and grill for another 4 or 5 minutes, or until chicken is no longer pink and the juices run clear. Or, grill on indoor grill, for 4 to 5 minutes, or until the chicken is no longer pink and the juices run clear. Serve over rice.

Divide and weigh each meal to assure the meals all weigh the same, within a few tenths of an ounce.

Dinner - 4 Blocks

Teriyaki Chicken with Fruit Salad for 3		P	C	F
12 oz.	Chicken Breasts, skinless, boneless	78.0	0	4.8
6 T	Teriyaki Marinade	6.0	18.0	0
1½ C	White Rice, cooked	6.0	57.0	0
1 C	Broccoli	3.0	6.0	0.5
1½ C	Cauliflower	3.0	7.5	0
3 T	Butter	0	0	33.0
Fruit Salad:				
¼ C	Mandarin Oranges, light	0.5	8.0	0
1½ C	Strawberries, sliced	1.5	10.5	0
15	Grapes	0	7.5	0
1 T	Mandarin Orange Salad Dressing	0	3.0	1.1
		98.0	117.5	39.4
		14.0	13.0	13.1
		4.6	4.3	4.3

Mandarin Orange Salad Dressing:
1 t	Canola Oil
3 T	Mandarin Orange liquid, light
1 t	Red Wine Vinegar
1 t	Cider Vinegar
1 t	Sugar

Teriyaki Marinade: Makes 2/3 Cups
¼ C	Light Brown Sugar packed.
¼ C	Soy Sauce
2 T	Lemon Juice
1 T	Canola oil
¼ t	Ground Ginger
¼ t	Garlic, minced

Prepare rice as directed on package but omit the butter.

Place chicken breasts in a large resealable bag. Make the Teriyaki marinade, pour over the chicken and seal the bag. Turn bag occasionally to make sure the chicken is coated all over. Refrigerate for 3 to 6 hours. (You will be making about 2/3 Cup of Teriyaki mix, but, after marinating, you will have used only about 2 Tablespoons.)

Discard leftover marinade. Grill chicken on grill 4 to 5 minutes, turn and grill another 4 to 5 minutes, or until the chicken is no longer pink and the juices run clear.

(You can omit the Mandarin Oranges, and still be balanced.)

Divide and weigh each meal to assure the meals all weigh the same, within a few tenths of an ounce.

Dinner - 5 Blocks

Chicken Cordon Bleu for 3

		P	C	F
12 oz.	Chicken Breasts, skinless boneless (4 oz. ea.)	78.0	0	4.8
2 T	White Flour	1.4	11.0	0
1 t	Paprika	0	0	0
2½ T	Butter	0	0	27.5
-	Fat Free Cooking Spray	0	0	0
3 slices	Swiss Cheese, fat free	15.0	6.0	0
3 slices	Honey Ham Deli-Thin 97% lean	5.0	1.0	0.7
½ C	White Wine	0	0	0
2	Chicken Bouillon Cubes	0	2.0	0
1 T	Corn Starch	0	7.0	0
1 C	Milk 2%	8.0	11.0	5.0
8	Red Potatoes, small (16 oz. peeled)	4.0	28.0	0
¼ C	Cheddar Cheese, fat free, grated	8.0	1.0	1.5
2 T	Green Onions, chopped	0	0.6	0
1 T	Butter	0	0	11.0
1 can	Green Beans (14.5 oz.)	1.5	7.0	0
2	Tangerines	0	18.0	0
1½ C	Strawberries, diced	1.5	10.5	0
1½ C	Cool Whip, fat free	0	48.0	0
		122.4	151.1	50.5
		17.4	16.7	16.8
		5.8	5.5	5.6

Place chicken breasts between 2 pieces of wax paper and lightly pound to flatten. Spread flattened chicken breasts, roll ham and cheese together, jellyroll style, and place in center of the chicken breasts. Fold breasts over and fasten with toothpicks. Mix flour and paprika and coat chicken breasts.

Spray skillet with fat free cooking spray; add 2½ Tablespoons of butter and heat. Add chicken and cook, turning until all sides are lightly brown. Add wine and bouillon. Reduce heat to low, cover and simmer until chicken is no longer pink. Remove chicken; pull out the toothpicks and cover to keep warm.

Mix cornstarch and milk. Add to the drippings in pan and stir until mixture thickens. Return the chicken to the pan and heat. Place chicken on the plates, divide the gravy and pour over the chicken.

While chicken is cooking, peel potatoes, dice and steam. Mash the potatoes; stir in cheddar cheese, green onions, and 1 Tablespoon of butter. Keep warm until ready to serve. Heat the green beans.

Divide and weigh each meal to assure the meals all weigh the same, within a few tenths of an ounce.

Dinner - 4 Blocks

Chicken Diane for 3		P	C	F
12 oz.	Chicken Breasts, skinless, boneless	78.0	0	4.8
-	Salt & pepper	0	0	0
-	Fat Free Cooking Spray	0	0	0
½ T	Lemon Juice	0	0.5	0
2 T	Green Onions, chopped	0.3	0.6	0
2 T	Red Wine	0	0	0
1 T	Parsley, fresh, chopped	0	1.0	0
2 t	Dijon mustard	0	0	0
1 can	Green Beans	1.5	7.0	0
3	Corn on Cob, medium ear	12.0	84.0	0
3 T	Butter	0	0	33.0
Salad:				
2 C	Romaine Lettuce	6.0	10.0	0
½	Tomato, medium	0.5	3.0	0
2 T	Green Onions	0.2	0.6	0
½ oz.	Cheddar Cheese, fat free	4.0	0.5	0
3 T	Thousand Island Dressing, fat free	0	12.0	0
		102.5	119.2	37.8
		14.6	13.2	12.6
		4.8	4.4	4.2

Place chicken breasts between 2 sheets of wax paper and pound lightly. Sprinkle with salt and pepper. Spray a cool skillet with fat free cooking spray and add the oil. Heat.

Cook chicken over medium high heat, no longer than 4 minutes on each side. Remove chicken and add green onions, lemon juice, red wine, parsley and mustard. Cook for about 15 seconds. Return chicken to skillet and heat.

Steam corn. Use 1 Tablespoon of butter on each ear of corn. Heat green beans. Serve with salad.

Divide the lettuce, dice tomatoes and green onions, and place in a large bowl. Add the salad dressing and mix well. Slice cheese in very small pieces. Divide the salad into 3 bowls then divide the cheese pieces and place on each salad. (Or try another fat free salad dressing that has about the same number of carbohydrates.)

Divide and weigh each meal to assure the meals all weigh the same, within a few tenths of an ounce.

Dinner - 4 Blocks

Chicken Bruschetta for 3

		P	C	F
12 oz.	Chicken Breasts, skinless, boneless	78.0	0	4.8
-	Fat Free Cooking Spray	0	0	0
½ t	Salt, divided	0	0	0
¼ t	Black pepper, divided	0	0	0
1 t	Garlic powder	0	0	0
1½ T	Olive oil	0	0	21.0
1 C	Zucchini, small, quartered lengthwise	2.0	4.0	0
8 oz.	Mushrooms, sliced	1.4	2.2	0.4
4	Garlic cloves minced	0	0	0
1 C	Tomatoes, chopped	1.6	6.0	0.6
½ C	Red onion, chopped	0.9	3.6	0.1
½ C	Basil, fresh chopped	0	0	0
4 t	Balsamic vinegar	0	0.9	0
¼ C	Parmesan cheese, fat free	0	18.0	0
1 C	White Rice, cooked	4.0	38.0	0

Mandarin Orange Salad:

1 C	Romaine Lettuce	3.0	5.0	0
¼ C	Mandarin Oranges, light	0.5	8.0	0
30	Grapes	0	15.0	0
1 C	Strawberries, sliced	1.0	7.0	0
1 T	Mandarin Orange Salad Dressing	0	3.0	1.1
1 T	Almonds, slivered	3.0	3.0	8.0
		95.4	113.7	36.0
		13.6	12.6	12.0
		4.5	4.2	4.0

Mandarin Orange Salad Dressing: Makes 4 Tablespoons.

1 t	Canola Oil
3 T	Mandarin Orange liquid, light
1 t	Red Wine Vinegar
1 t	Cider Vinegar
1 t	Sugar

Prepare rice as directed on package but omit the butter.

Heat grill. Prepare rice according to the package directions but omit butter.
Combine garlic powder, half the salt and pepper in a small bowl, sprinkle chicken with garlic powder mixture. Grill chicken until the chicken is no longer pink and the juices run clear. Divide rice by 3 on each plate. Lay grilled chicken on top of rice.

Spray a cool skillet with fat free cooking spray. Add the oil and fry over medium-high heat. Add rest of salt, mushrooms, zucchini, and minced garlic, sauté 2 minutes. Add the remaining pepper, salt, tomato, onion, basil, and vinegar sauté 3 minutes. Place 1/3 of the rice on each plate. Serve the vegetable mixture over the chicken. Sprinkle with cheese.

Divide and weigh each meal to assure the meals all weigh the same, within a few tenths of an ounce.

Dinner - 4 Blocks

Chicken Stir-Fry for 3

		P	C	F
10.5 oz.	Chicken Breasts, skinless, boneless	68.2	0	4.2
1 T	Olive Oil	0	0	14.0
3 T	Chicken Broth	0	0	0
½ C	Green Pepper, diced	0.4	5.6	0.1
½ C	Onions, diced	0.9	5.6	0.1
½ C	Snow Peas	2.0	6.0	0
½ C	Carrots	1.0	11.5	0
1 C	Cauliflower	2.0	5.0	0
1 C	Broccoli	3.0	6.0	0
¼ C	Stir-Fry Sauce	0	12.0	0
6 T	Soy Sauce	6.0	6.0	0
1½ C	White Rice, cooked	6.0	57.0	0
2 oz.	Cashews (28 lg. or 52 sm.)	10.0	16.0	26.0
		99.8	130.7	44.4
		14.2	14.5	14.8
		4.7	4.8	4.9

Prepare rice as directed on package but omit the butter.

Cut chicken breasts crosswise, into ¼" wide strips. Spray a cool wok with fat free cooking spray; add the olive oil and heat. Stir in carrots, cauliflower and broccoli. Cook until vegetables are crisp-tender. (About 5 minutes)

Add onion, green pepper and snow peas. Cook another 3 minutes. Remove vegetables to a warm bowl and add the chicken strips to the wok. Stir fry chicken until no longer pink and the juices run clear. (About 5 minutes)

Return vegetables to the skillet. In a cup, mix cornstarch with 2 T of soy sauce until smooth. Gradually add mixture to the wok and cook, stirring until mixture thickens. Add Stir-Fry Sauce and heat.

When ready to serve, divide rice and put on plate. Divide the chicken stir-fry as close as possible and put on top of the rice. Divide the cashews and put on each plate.

Divide and weigh each meal to assure the meals all weigh the same, within a few tenths of an ounce.

Dinner - 4 Blocks

Mushroom-Garlic Chicken With Artichokes for 3

		P	C	F
10.5 oz.	Chicken Breasts, skinless, boneless	68.2	0	4.2
1 C	Mushrooms, sliced	2.0	4.0	0
12 oz.	Artichoke Hearts, canned	11.7	34.2	0.6
2 T	Marsala Wine	0	2.0	0
1 T	Lemon Juice	0	0	0
3 T	Butter	0	0	33.0
8	Garlic Cloves, pressed	0	0	0
1½ C	White Rice, cooked	6.0	57.0	0
-	Salt & freshly ground pepper	0	0	0
4 C	Romaine Lettuce	12.0	20.0	0
¼ C	Mandarin Oranges, light	0.5	8.0	0
10	Grapes	0	5.0	0
3 T	Mandarin Orange Salad Dressing	0	0.6	3.4
		100.4	128.8	41.2
		14.3	14.3	13.7
		4.7	4.7	4.5

Mandarin Orange Salad Dressing: Makes 4 Tablespoons.

1 t	Canola Oil
3 T	Mandarin Orange liquid, light
1 t	Red Wine Vinegar
1 t	Cider Vinegar
1 t	Sugar

Prepare rice as directed on package but omit the butter.

Season chicken with salt and pepper and set aside.

Spray a cool skillet with fat free cooking spray; add 2 T butter and heat. Add half the garlic and cook 1 minute. Add the seasoned chicken and cook until lightly brown, about 3 minutes a side. Remove the chicken from the skillet and keep warm.

In the same skillet, add 1 T of butter and remaining garlic: cook 1 minute. Add the mushrooms and cook until tender, About 3 minutes.) Add artichokes and cook until heated through. Add Marsala wine and lemon juice. Bring to a boil, stirring continuously until mixture thickens, about 5 minutes

Divide and weigh each meal to assure the meals all weigh about the same, within a few tenths of an ounce.

Dinner - 4 Blocks

Chicken Dijon with Ginger Pear Sauce for 3		P	C	F
12 oz.	Chicken Breasts, skinless, boneless	78.0	0	4.8
-	Fat Free Cooking Spray	0	0	0
2 T	Butter	0	0	22.0
-	Salt and Pepper to taste	0	0	0
15½ oz	Pears, sliced, in juice	1.9	52.5	0
½ C	Green Onions, thinly sliced	1.0	2.4	0
1 T	Molasses	0	15.0	0
1 t	Ginger Root	0	0	0
½ T	Dijon Mustard	0	0	0
½ C	Snow Peas, raw	2.0	6.0	0
2 t	Butter	0	0	7.2
1 C	Romaine Lettuce	3.0	5.0	0
1 C	Strawberries, sliced	1.0	7.0	0
30	Grapes	0	15.0	0
1 T	Mandarin Orange Salad Dressing	0	3.0	1.1
		86.9	105.9	35.1
		12.4	11.7	11.7
		4.1	3.9	3.9

Mandarin Orange Salad Dressing: Makes 4 Tablespoons.
1 t	Canola Oil
3 T	Mandarin Orange liquid, light
1 t	Red Wine Vinegar
1 t	Cider Vinegar
1 t	Sugar

Drain pears and reserve liquid. Set aside. Season chicken with salt and pepper.

Spray a cool skillet with fat free cooking spray; add 2 T butter and heat. Cook chicken, about 9 minutes, or until chicken is no longer pink. Remove to a platter.

Add reserved pear liquid, green onions, molasses, ginger and mustard to skillet. Bring to a boil, scraping browned bits from pan. Reduce the heat and cook for about 2 minutes. Return chicken to skillet; add pears and heat through. Place chicken on plates and spoon on the pear sauce.

Steam Snow Peas and melt 2 t Butter on top. Serve with salad.

Combine salad dressing ingredients, shake well and pour 1 Tablespoon over the lettuce. Mix well, divide and place in bowls. Cut the grapes in half. Divide mandarin oranges, grapes and strawberries. Place on top of the lettuce.

Divide and weigh each meal to assure the meals all weigh the same, within a few tenths of an ounce.

Dinner - 4 Blocks

Orange Chicken with Green Grapes for 3

		P	C	F
12 oz.	Chicken Breasts, skinless, boneless	78.0	0	4.8
-	Fat Free Cooking Spray	0	0	0
1 T	Butter	0	0	11.0
-	Salt and Pepper to taste	0	0	0
¼ t	Paprika	0	0	0
½ C	Orange Juice	2.0	26.0	0
1 T	Green Onions, chopped	0	0	0
1	Chicken Bouillon Cube	0	1.0	0
1 T	Cornstarch	0	7.0	0
30	Green Grapes, seedless, halved	0	15.0	0
11 oz.	Corn (canned)	8.0	40.0	2.0
1 T	Butter	0	0	11.0
8	Red Potatoes, small (16 oz. peeled)	4.0	28.0	0
¼ C	Cheddar Cheese, fat free, grated	8.0	1.0	1.5
2 T	Green Onions, chopped	0	0.6	0
1 T	Butter	0	0	11.0
		100.0	118.6	41.3
		14.2	13.1	13.1
		4.7	4.3	4.3

Spray a cool skillet with fat free cooking spray and brown chicken on all sides.

Preheat oven to 350 degrees. Arrange chicken in a 13 x 9 x 2 Baking pan. Season with salt, pepper and paprika.

In a small bowl mix together orange juice, green onions, and bouillon cube. Pour mixture over chicken and bake until the chicken is no longer pink and the juices run clear. Remove chicken and place on a platter and keep warm.
Dissolved the cornstarch in 1 T of water and stir into pan drippings and bring to a boil. Cook until thick and bubbly, stirring constantly. Add grapes and cook until hot.

While chicken is cooking, peel potatoes, dice and steam. Mash the potatoes; stir in cheddar cheese, green onions, and 1 Tablespoon of butter. Keep warm until ready to serve. Heat the corn and melt 1 T of butter over the top before serving.

Divide and weigh each meal to assure the meals all weigh the same, within a few tenths of an ounce.

Dinner - 4 Blocks

	Grilled Chicken-Vegetable Packets for 3	P	C	F
12 oz.	Chicken Breasts (3 breasts, 4 oz. each)	78.0	0	4.8
-	Fat Free Cooking Spray	0	0	0
1 med.	Zucchini, cut into ½-inch slices	0.3	0.3	0
6	Potatoes, New Red, small (12 oz.)	4.0	27.8	0
1 C	Carrots, cut in chunks	2.0	23.0	0
-	Salt and Pepper to taste	0	0	0
1 C	Mushrooms, sliced	0.6	0.9	0.1
6	Pearl Onions	0.6	7.5	0
2 T	Butter	0	0	22.0
½ C	Water	0	0	0
3 slices	Wheat Bread, Pepperidge Farm, light	7.0	22.0	1.0
1 T	Butter	0	0	11.0
3	Plums	0	27.0	0
		92.5	108.5	39.8
		13.2	12.0	13.2
		4.4	4.0	4.4

Tear off 3 pieces of aluminum foil (about 18" square.) Spray the foil with fat free cooking spray.

Add 1 piece of chicken breast to each. Divide zucchini, potatoes, carrots mushrooms and onions and place on top of chicken. Sprinkle about 4 tablespoons of water over vegetables. Place 1 Tablespoon of butter on top of each and season with salt and pepper to taste.

Seal foil into packets, leaving room for steam. Grill over medium coals for 30 to 25 minutes, or until chicken is done and vegetables are tender, turning once.

Serve with 1 slice of bread each with 1 teaspoon of butter. Have a plum, tangerine, or peach for dessert.

Divide and weigh each meal to assure the meals all weigh the same, within a few tenths of an ounce.

Dinner - 4 Blocks

Coq au Vin Blanc (Chicken with White Wine) for 3

		P	C	F
12 oz.	Chicken Breasts, skinless, boneless	78.0	0	4.8
-	Salt, to taste	0	0	0
-	White Pepper to taste	0	0	0
½ C	White Wine	0	0	0
1 t	Garlic, chopped	0	0	0
½ t	Thyme leaves, dried	0	0	0
2 T	White Flour	1.5	11.0	0
-	Fat Free Cooking Spray	0	0	0
2 ½ T	Canola Oil	0	0	35.0
-	Plastic Food Storage Bag	0	0	0
10	Red Potatoes, small (20 oz. peeled)	6.0	35.0	0
1 C	Carrots, raw, diced	2.0	23.0	0
½ C	Onions, chopped	0.9	5.6	0.1
4 oz.	Baby Mushrooms	2.5	3.3	0.5
5 oz.	Red Pearl Onions	0.6	4.0	0
¼ C	Chicken Broth	0	0	0
1 t	Tomato Paste	0	0	0
1 t	Dijon Mustard	0	0	0
1	Bay Leaf	0	0	0
1 T	Parsley, freshly chopped	0	1.0	0
1½ C	Strawberries, diced	1.5	10.5	0
1 C	Cool Whip, fat free	0	32.0	0
		93.0	125.4	40.4
		13.2	13.9	13.4
		4.4	4.6	4.4

Season both sides of chicken with salt and pepper. Arrange chicken in a baking dish; add wine, garlic and thyme to chicken. Marinate for 45 minutes. Remove chicken from marinade, reserving marinade. Drain on paper towels; place in food storage bag with flour. Shake to coat. Remove chicken from bag and tap off excess flour. In saucepan or Dutch oven, heat oil over medium-high heat. Sauté chicken until golden brown on all sides. (About 5 minutes per side.) Remove chicken. Stir in potatoes and carrots and cook 5 minutes. Stir in pearl onions, mushrooms and chopped onions, cook 2 minutes. Add reserved marinade, broth, tomato paste, mustard and bay leaf. Return chicken to pan, stirring to coat chicken with sauce.

To serve: Arrange chicken pieces in a serving dish, pour sauce over the top and sprinkle with parsley.

Serve Strawberries and Cool Whip for dessert.

Dinner - 4 Blocks

Sesame Chicken for 3

		P	C	F
12 oz.	Chicken Breasts, skinless, boneless	78.0	0	4.8
-	Fat Free Cooking Spray	0	0	0
1 T	Sesame Seeds	1.6	2.0	4.4
1 T	Sesame Oil	0	0	13.6
1½ T	Canola Oil	0	0	21.0
1 T	Soy Sauce	2.0	0	0
1	Green Pepper, seeded, cut into strips	0.7	3.0	0
1 C	Snow Peas	4.0	12.0	0
½ C	Carrots, sliced thinly	1.0	11.5	0
4	Scallions, diagonal chopped	0.3	0.9	0.1
1 C	Pineapple, diced, light	1.0	32.0	0
1½ C	White Rice, cooked	6.0	57.0	0

Marinade:

2 t	Cornstarch	0	4.6	0
2 T	Chinese Rice Wine	0	0	0
1 T	Lemon Juice	0.1	1.3	0
2 drops	Tabasco Sauce	0	0	0
1'	Ginger Root, grated	0	0	0
1	Garlic Clove	0	0	0
		94.7	124.3	43.9
		13.5	13.8	14.6
		4.5	4.6	4.8

Prepare rice according to package directions but omit the butter.

Cut chicken into about ½ X 2". In a small bowl, mix the cornstarch with the rice wine then stir in lemon juice, soy sauce, Tabasco sauce, ginger and garlic. Add the chicken strips, cover and marinate for 3 to 4 hours.

Heat the Wok to medium and dry fry the sesame seeds, stirring, until the seeds are golden. Remove from the Wok and set aside. Add the Canola oil and Sesame oil and heat. Drain the chicken, reserving the marinade, and add the chicken to the Wok. Stir fry until brown. Remove from the Wok.

Add the green pepper, carrots and snow peas. Stir fry 2-3 minutes. Add the scallions and stir-fry for 1 minute more.

Return the chicken to the Wok; add the reserved marinade and stir over medium heat for about 2 minutes, or until ingredients are evenly coated with glaze. Sprinkle with sesame seeds and stir. Serve over rice.

Fish Dinner Choices

Dinner - 4 Blocks

Grilled Salmon Fillets with Wild Rice for 3		P	C	F
12 oz.	Salmon fillets, (1" thick)	90.0	0	27.0
-	Fat Free Cooking Spray	0	0	0
-	Salt and Pepper to taste	0	0	0
1 t	Olive Oil	0	0	4.6
¼ C	White Wine	0	0	0
2	Garlic Cloves, large, minced	0	0	0
¼ C	Parsley, fresh, snipped	0	0	0
¼ C	Chicken Broth	0	0	0
¼ t	Red Pepper, crushed	0	0	0
1 C	Wild Rice, (¼ C raw)	6.0	33.0	0.5
1 C	Cauliflower, raw	2.0	5.0	0
1 C	Carrots, sliced	2.0	23.0	0
1 T	Butter	0	0	11.0
Dessert:				
3 C	Peaches, fresh (2½" each)	0	27.0	0
1 C	Cool Whip, fat free	0	24.0	0
2 t	Sugar	0	4.0	0
		100.0	120.0	43.0
		14.2	13.3	14.3
		4.7	4.4	4.7

Sprinkle both sides of salmon with salt and pepper to taste. Shape a large piece of aluminum foil into a bowl; spray with fat free cooking spray. Place the salmon in the center.

Combine olive oil, wine, chicken broth, garlic and red pepper. Pour mixture over salmon. Seal the foil and marinate in the refrigerator for about 30 minutes.

While salmon is marinating, prepare rice. Follow directions on package, but don't add any butter.

When ready to prepare dinner, heat grill, open salmon packet and place on grill. Grill salmon, turning once, (8 to 10 minutes) or until the salmon flakes easily with a fork.

While salmon is grilling, prepare vegetables and steam until crisp tender. Melt butter over them.

Dessert:
Peel peaches, cut into slices and sprinkle with the sugar. Divide and serve with Whipped topping for dessert.

Divide and weigh each meal to assure the meals all weigh the same, within a few tenths of an ounce.

Dinner - 4 Blocks

Baked Salmon with Apple Glaze for 3   P   C   F

9 oz.	Salmon fillets, (1" thick)	67.5	0	20.2
-	Fat Free Cooking Spray	0	0	0
-	Salt and Pepper to taste	0	0	0
1 t	Thyme, fresh, finely chopped	0	0	0
1 t	Rosemary, fresh, finely chopped	0	0	0
¼ C	Vermouth	0	0.8	0
¼ C	Apple Jelly	0	48.0	0
1 C	Wild Rice, (¼ C raw)	6.0	33.0	0.5
1 C	Broccoli	3.0	6.0	0.5
4 t	Butter	0	0	14.6
1 C	Lettuce, leafy	3.0	5.0	0
1 C	Strawberries	1.0	7.0	0
15	Grapes	0	7.5	0
1 T	Mandarin Orange Salad Dressing	0	3.0	1.1
		80.5	107.3	36.9
		11.5	11.9	12.3
		3.8	3.9	4.1

Mandarin Orange Salad Dressing: Makes 4 Tablespoons.
- 1 t   Canola Oil
- 3 T   Mandarin Orange liquid, light
- 1 t   Red Wine Vinegar
- 1 t   Cider Vinegar
- 1 t   Sugar

Preheat oven to 400 degrees.

Apple Glaze:
In a small saucepan, place thyme, rosemary, and vermouth. Bring to a boil and stir in the apple jelly. Simmer, just until the jelly is melted. Remove from heat and set aside.

Salmon:
Spray a cool skillet with fat free cooking spray. Sprinkle salmon with salt and pepper to taste and cook, until lightly brown

Transfer salmon to a 2-quart baking dish. Pour the apple glaze over the salmon and bake for 8 to 10 minutes, or until the salmon flakes easily with a fork, and the glaze is lightly brown and caramelized. Serve over wild rice with green beans and a salad.

Divide and weigh each meal to assure the meals all weigh the same, within a few tenths of an ounce.

Dinner - 4 Blocks

Grilled Salmon with Lemon Rosemary Marinade for 3   P   C   F

		P	C	F
9 oz	Salmon Fillets (4 oz. each)	67.5	0	20.2
-	Fat Free Cooking Spray	0	0	0
¼ C	Rice, Wild, cooked (1C Cooked)	6.0	33.0	0.5
2 C	Zucchini, sliced	4.0	8.0	0
1 C	Onions, sliced	1.8	11.0	0
12	Asparagus Spears, fresh	4.8	4.8	4.8
1 t	Butter	0	0	3.6
1 C	Romaine Lettuce	3.0	5.0	0
3 C	Strawberries, sliced	3.0	21.0	0
30	Grapes	0	15.0	0
1 T	Almond, slivers	3.0	3.0	8.0
1 T	Mandarin Orange Salad Dressing	0	3.0	1.1
		93.1	103.8	38.2
		13.3	11.5	12.7
		4.4	3.8	4.2

Mandarin Orange Salad Dressing: Makes 4 Tablespoons.
1 t	Canola Oil
3 T	Mandarin Orange liquid, light
1 t	Red Wine Vinegar
1 t	Cider Vinegar
1 t	Sugar

Lemon Rosemary Marinade:
2 T	Canola Oil
2 T	Lemon Juice
¼	Green Onions, sliced
2 T	Fresh Parsley, chopped
½ t	Rosemary, dried
½ t	Salt
1/8 t	Pepper, freshly ground

    Prepare rice according to the recipe on the package. Do not use butter.
    Combine Marinade and mix well. Put salmon into a resealable bag. Reserve ¼ cup of the marinade. Pour the rest of the marinade over the salmon, seal the bag and refrigerate for about 1 hour, or until ready to grill. When ready, remove salmon from marinade, (discard marinade) and grill salmon over medium heat for 4 or 5 minutes. Turn, brush with reserve marinade and grill again for 4 or 5 minutes. Keep turning until fish flakes easily with a fork.
    Meanwhile, prepare vegetables and fry in the butter until crisp tender. Make the salad.
    Divide and weigh each meal to assure the meals all weigh the same, within a few tenths of an ounce.

Dinner - 4 Blocks

Grilled Swordfish with Mustard Sauce for 3   P   C   F

		P	C	F
12 oz	Swordfish Stakes (4 oz. each)	66.0	0	3.0
2 T	Lemon Juice	0	2.0	0
-	Savory Sauce	1.0	3.0	22.5
10	Potatoes, New Red, 2.5" (20 oz.)	6.6	46.6	0
1 C	Carrots, diced	2.0	23.0	0
1 T	Butter	0	0	11.0
1 C	Romaine Lettuce	3.0	5.0	0
2 C	Strawberries, sliced	2.0	14.0	1.2
30	Grapes	0	15.0	0
1 T	Mandarin Orange Salad Dressing	0	3.0	1.1
		80.6	111.6	38.8
		11.5	12.4	12.9
		3.8	4.1	4.3

Mandarin Orange Salad Dressing: Makes 4 Tablespoons.

1 t	Vegetable Oil
2 T	Mandarin Orange liquid, light
1 t	Red Wine Vinegar
1 t	Cider Vinegar
1 t	Sugar

Mustard Sauce:

2 T	Butter, melted
2 T	Dijon Mustard
1 T	Chili Sauce
1 T	Soy Sauce
1 T	Celery, diced

    Make the sauce and set aside. Heat grill. Brush tuna steaks with lemon juice, grill for 4 or 5 minutes. Turn and brush with mustard sauce. Continue brushing and turning until fish flakes easily with a fork. (Using up all the sauce)

    Meanwhile, steam vegetables. When ready to serve, melt butter over the top.

    Divide and weigh each meal to assure the meals all weigh the same, within a few tenths of an ounce.

Dinner - 4 Blocks

Grilled Tuna Steak with Ginger Lime Marinade for 3   P   C   F

9 oz	Tuna Steak, Blue Fin (3 oz. each)	59.4	0	12.6
2 T	Lime Juice	0	2.0	0
10	Potatoes, New Red, 2.5" (20 oz.)	6.6	46.6	0
1 C	Carrots, diced	2.0	23.0	0
1 T	Butter	0	0	11.0
1 C	Romaine Lettuce	3.0	5.0	0
2 C	Strawberries, sliced	2.0	14.0	0
30	Grapes	0	15.0	0
2 T	Almond slivers	4.5	4.5	12.0
1 T	Mandarin Orange Salad Dressing	0	3.0	1.1
		77.5	113.1	36.7
		11.0	12.5	12.2
		3.7	4.1	4.0

Mandarin Orange Salad Dressing: Makes 4 Tablespoons of dressing.

1 t	Canola Oil
2 T	Mandarin Orange liquid, light
1 t	Red Wine Vinegar
1 t	Cider Vinegar
1 t	Sugar

Ginger Lime Marinade:

2 T	Lime Juice
2 T	Liquid from Mandarin Orange light can
1 t	Ginger Root
-	Salt to taste
-	Cayenne Pepper
1	Garlic, Clove

    Make the ginger lime marinade and pour into a resealable food storage bag. Add the tuna, turning to coat and place into the refrigerator to marinate 1 to 3 hours. When ready to grill, remove tuna steaks to the grill.

    Save the marinade in a bowl to baste the tuna as it grills. Heat grill. Brush tuna steaks with lime juice and grill for 4 or 5 minutes. Turn and brush with the ginger lime marinade. Continue brushing and turning until fish flakes easily with a fork.

Meanwhile, steam vegetables. When ready to serve, melt butter over the top.

Divide and weigh each meal to assure the meals all weigh the same, within a few tenths of an ounce.

Dinner - 5 Blocks

Grilled Salmon with Lemon-Dill Mayonnaise for 3		P	C	F
9 oz	Salmon Steak (3 oz. each)	90.0	0	27.0
1 T	Lemon Juice	0	1.0	0
-	Lemon-Dill Mayonnaise	4.4	14.7	0
1 C	Cauliflower, raw	2.0	5.0	0
½ C	Snow Peas, raw	2.0	6.0	0
2 T	Butter	0	0	22.0
3 slices	1/12th Angel Food Cake	9.0	90.0	0
1½ C	Strawberries, sliced	1.5	10.5	0
6 T	Cool Whip, fat free	0	9.0	0
		108.9	136.2	49.0
		15.5	15.1	16.3
		5.1	5.0	5.4

Lemon-Dill Mayonnaise:
4 T	Miracle Whip, fat free
½ T	Fresh Parsley, snipped
1 T	Fresh Dill, snipped
½ t	Lemon Zest
1 t	Lemon Juice
1	Garlic Clove, small, minced
2 T	Buttermilk

Bake an Angel Food Cake mix. Divide into 12 equal pieces. The extra pieces can be frozen, or try one of the other recipes that serve Angel Food Cake, strawberries and/or fat free Cool Whip for dessert.

Place all ingredients in a blender and blend until smooth. Set aside.

Heat grill. Place the salmon on a piece of heavy-duty foil. Brush salmon with lemon juice and sprinkle with pepper. Seal the foil around the salmon. Place the foil packet on the grill and cover with the lid. Grill the salmon 4 to 6 inches from medium heat about 20 minutes, or until salmon flakes easily with a fork. When salmon is ready to serve place 1/3 of dill butter on top of each salmon steak and serve.

While the salmon is cooking steam vegetables and melt the butter over the top.

Serve angel food cake with strawberries and whip cream for dessert.

Divide and weigh each meal to assure the meals all weigh the same, within a few tenths of an ounce.

Dinner -5 Blocks

Grilled Salmon Steaks with Blue Cheese Crumbles for 3		P	C	F
9 oz	Salmon Steak (3 oz. each)	90.0	0	27.0
-	Fat Free Cooking Spray	0	0	0
1 T	Lemon Juice	0	1.0	0
1 oz	Blue Cheese Crumbles	1.8	0.2	2.4
1 C	Brussels Sprouts	6.0	20.0	1.0
1 C	Cauliflower, raw	2.0	5.0	0
½ C	Snow Peas, raw	2.0	6.0	0
2 T	Butter	0	0	22.0
3 slices	1/12th Angel Food Cake	9.0	90.0	0
1½ C	Strawberries, sliced	1.5	10.5	0
6 T	Cool Whip, fat free	0	9.0	0
		112.3	141.7	52.4
		16.0	15.7	17.4
		5.3	5.2	5.8

Bake an Angel Food Cake mix. Divide into 12 equal pieces. The extra pieces can be frozen, or try one of the other recipes that serve Angel Food Cake, strawberries and/or fat free Cool Whip for dessert.

Heat grill. Spray a piece of heavy-duty foil with fat free cooking spray. Place the salmon on a foil. Brush the salmon steaks with lemon juice and sprinkle with pepper. Seal the foil around the salmon.
Place the foil packet on the grill and cover with the lid. Grill the salmon 4 to 6 inches from medium heat about 20 minutes, or until salmon flakes easily with a fork.

Meanwhile, steam vegetables and melt the butter over the top.

Serve angel food cake with strawberries and whip cream for dessert.

Divide and weigh each meal to assure the meals all weigh the same, within a few tenths of an ounce.

Dinner - 4 Blocks

Fish and Chips for 3   P   C   F

		P	C	F
15 oz.	Orange Roughy (or any other white fish)	60.0	0	3.7
-	Fat Free Cooking Spray	0	0	0
2 T	Butter	0	0	22.0
2 T	Wheat Germ, toasted	4.0	4.0	1.0
2 T	Bread Crumbs, plain	2.0	9.0	0.7
-	Salt	0	0	0
-	Ground Red Pepper (Cayenne) (pinch)	0	0	0
½ T	Dijon Mustard	0	0	0
3	Lemon wedges	0	1.0	0
-	Non-Stick Spray	0	0	0
4	Red Potatoes, (about 24 oz.)	7.7	55.7	0
-	Salt and Pepper to taste	0	0	0

Mandarin Orange Salad:

2 C	Romaine Lettuce	6.0	10.0	0
¼ C	Mandarin Oranges, light	0.5	8.0	0
10	Grapes	0	5.0	0
1 C	Strawberries, sliced	1.0	7.0	0
1 T	Almonds, slivered	3.0	3.0	8.0
2 T	Mandarin Orange Salad Dressing	0	6.0	2.2
		84.2	108.7	37.6
		12.0	12.0	12.5
		4.0	4.0	4.1

Mandarin Orange Salad Dressing:

- 1 t   Canola Oil
- 3 T   Mandarin Orange liquid, light
- 1 t   Red Wine Vinegar
- 1 t   Cider Vinegar
- 1 t   Sugar

Preheat oven to 500 degrees. Spray 2 large cookie sheets with fat free cooking spray. Wash potatoes, cut out eyes and slice to ¼" thick.

Place potatoes in a bowl and toss with the salt and pepper. Divide potato slices evenly between pans. Bake about 20 minutes or until tender and lightly browned.

Fish:

Combine wheat germ, breadcrumbs, salt, and ground red pepper. Lightly brush sides with mustard then coat with the wheat germ mixture.

Spray non-stick skillet with non-stick spray. Heat skillet over medium-high heat and cook the fish for about 5 minutes on each side or until fish flakes easily when tested with a fork and coating is golden brown. Serve with lemon wedges.

Divide and weigh each meal to assure the meals all weigh the same, within a few tenths of an ounce.

Dinner - 4 Blocks

Shrimp Scampi for 3   P   C   F

		P	C	F
12 oz.	Shrimp, large, (about 12 each)	72.0	0	4.8
-	Fat Free Cooking Spray	0	0	0
2 T	Butter	0	0	22.0
¼ C	White Wine	0	0	0
5	Garlic Cloves, minced	0	0	0
-	Salt and freshly ground Pepper to taste	0	0	0
1 t	Parsley	0	0	0
3 oz.	Angel Hair Spaghetti	10.0	79.9	1.9
1 oz.	Feta Cheese, crumbled	4.0	1.2	6.0

Mandarin Orange Salad:

		P	C	F
2 C	Romaine Lettuce	6.0	10.0	0
¼ C	Mandarin Oranges, light	0.5	8.0	0
15	Grapes	0	7.5	0
1½ C	Strawberries, diced	1.5	10.5	0
½ T	Almonds, thinly sliced	1.5	1.5	4.0
1 T	Mandarin Orange Salad Dressing	0	3.0	1.1
		95.5	121.6	39.8
		13.6	13.5	13.2
		4.5	4.5	4.4

Mandarin Orange Salad Dressing: Makes 4 Tablespoons.
- 1 t   Canola Oil
- 3 T   Mandarin Orange liquid, light
- 1 t   Red Wine Vinegar
- 1 t   Cider Vinegar
- 1 t   Sugar

Spray a cool skillet with fat free cooking spray fat free cooking spray. Add the butter, salt, and garlic. Heat over low heat for a few minutes. Raise the heat to medium and add the shrimp. When the shrimp turns pink on one side, turn it over and cook about 2 minutes more. Add the white wine and cook another 30 seconds. Garnish with parsley. Cook spaghetti and add to the skillet, stirring to coat. Heat until warm. Divide shrimp (about 12 each) and spaghetti. Sprinkle with Feta Cheese and freshly ground pepper.

Prepare the lettuce. Combine salad dressing ingredients, shake well and pour 1 Tablespoon over the lettuce. Mix well. Divide lettuce and put in bowls. Cut grapes in half. Dice the strawberries. Divide the grapes, strawberries and mandarin oranges and place on top of lettuce. Sprinkle almonds on top.

(You can omit the mandarin oranges and grapes, or the strawberries, and still have a balanced meal.)

Divide and weigh each meal to assure the meals all weigh the same, within a few tenths of an ounce.

Dinner - 5 Blocks

Salmon Patties for 3		P	C	F
14¾ oz. can	Pink Salmon	84.6	0	30.0
1	Egg, whole	6.0	0	5.0
¼ C	Onions, diced	0.4	2.8	0
1 slice	Wheat Bread, Pepperidge Farm, light	2.0	7.0	0
-	Salt and Pepper to taste	0	0	0
-	Fat Free Cooking Spray	0	0	0
-	White Sauce	4.7	11.5	2.5
1 C	Cauliflower	2.0	5.0	0
1 C	Broccoli	3.0	6.0	0.5
1 T	Butter	0	0	11.0
Dessert:				
3 slices	1/12th Angel Food Cake	9.0	93.0	0
1½ C	Strawberries, sliced	1.5	10.5	0
6 T	Cool Whip, fat free	0	9.0	0
		113.2	144.8	49.0
		16.1	16.0	16.3
		5.3	5.3	5.4

White Sauce:
3 T	Water
1 T	Cornstarch
½ C	Milk, 2%
-	Salt, Paprika and Pepper to taste

Bake an Angel Food Cake mix. Divide into 12 equal pieces. The extra pieces can be frozen, or try one of the other recipes that serve Angel Food Cake, strawberries and fat free whipped topping for dessert.

Drain the liquid from the salmon. In a large bowl, place the salmon, egg, diced onions, bread crumbs, and salt and pepper to taste. Shape salmon mixture into 3 equal sized patties. Spray a cool skillet with fat free cooking spray and heat. Fry salmon patties until lightly brown. While the salmon patties are browning, make the white sauce. Stir the cornstarch into the milk, add the rest of the ingredients in a small saucepan, heat and stir over medium heat until thickened. Do not boil.

Steam vegetables and melt the butter over the top. Stir. Divide vegetables by 3 and place on each plate.

When ready to serve, put salmon patties on the plate and pour the white sauce evenly over them. Serve with angel food cake, strawberries and fat free whipped topping. (You can omit the cool whip and still have a balanced meal.)

Divide and weigh each meal to assure the meals all weigh the same, within a few tenths of an ounce.

Dinner - 4 Blocks

Grilled Halibut for 3   P   C   F

12 oz.	Halibut Fillets (or any other white fish)	48.0	0	3.0
-	Fat Free Cooking Spray	0	0	0
1 T	Butter	0	0	11.0
3 T	Heinz Ketchup	0	12.0	0
11 oz.	Corn (canned)	8.0	40.0	2.0
1 can	Asparagus (15 oz.)	7.0	7.0	0
1 T	Butter	0	0	11.0
24 oz.	Milk, 2% (8 oz. each)	24.0	33.0	15.0

Mandarin Orange Salad:

1 C	Romaine Lettuce	3.0	5.0	0
20	Grapes	0	10.0	0
1 C	Strawberries, sliced	1.0	7.0	0
1 t	Sugar	0	4.0	0
1 T	Mandarin Orange Salad Dressing	0	3.0	1.1
		91.0	121.0	41.1
		13.0	13.4	13.7
		4.3	4.4	4.5

Mandarin Orange Salad Dressing: Makes 4 Tablespoons.

1 t	Canola Oil
3 T	Mandarin Orange liquid, light
1 t	Red Wine Vinegar
1 t	Cider Vinegar
1 t	Sugar

Thaw fish in a few Tablespoons of milk until ready to cook. Discard the left over milk. Sprinkle fish with salt and pepper and fry or grill until the fish flakes. While the fish is grilling, heat the vegetables and put ½ T of butter on each. Divide by 3 and serve.

You can substitute 5 T of fat free Miracle Whip for the 3 Tablespoons of ketchup (or a combination) and still be balanced.

Combine salad dressing ingredients, shake well and pour 1 Tablespoon of dressing over the lettuce, mix well, divide and place in bowls. Cut Grapes in half. Chop strawberries. Divide strawberries and grapes, and place on top of lettuce.

(You can omit strawberries and grapes and still have a balanced meal.)

Divide and weigh each meal to assure the meals all weigh the same, within a few tenths of an ounce.

Dinner - 4 Blocks

	Cheesy Orange Roughy for 3	P	C	F
12 oz.	Orange Roughy (or any other white fish)	64.0	0	4.0
3 T	Parmesan Cheese, fat free	4.5	13.5	0
-	Fat Free Cooking Spray	0	0	0
1 T	Butter	0	0	11.0
6 T	Heinz Ketchup	0	24.0	0
1 C	Brussels Sprouts	6.0	20.0	1.0
1 C	Cauliflower	2.0	5.0	0
1 T	Butter	0	0	11.0
	Mandarin Orange Salad:			
3 C	Romaine Lettuce	9.0	15.0	0
¼ C	Mandarin Oranges, light	0.5	8.0	0
15	Grapes	0	7.5	0
1 C	Strawberries, sliced	1.0	7.0	0
1 T	Almond slivered	3.0	3.0	8.0
2 T	Mandarin Orange Salad Dressing	0	6.0	2.2
		90.0	109.0	37.2
		12.8	12.1	12.4
		4.2	4.0	4.1

Thaw fish in milk. Discard the left over milk. Spray a cool skillet with fat free cooking spray and add 1 Tablespoon of butter. Heat skillet, sprinkle the fish with salt and pepper and fry fish until it flakes, (7 to 10 min.) Sprinkle Parmesan cheese over fish, cover and keep warm.

Steam Brussels sprouts and cauliflower. Melt butter over top, divide and serve.

Combine salad dressing ingredients, shake well and pour 2 Tablespoons of dressing over the lettuce, mix well, divide and place in bowls. Cut grapes in half. Dice strawberries. Divide mandarin oranges, strawberries and grapes and place on top of lettuce.

(You can omit strawberries or grapes and still have a balanced meal.)

(You can omit ketchup and add 16 Tablespoons of Miracle Whip, fat free and still be balanced.)

Divide and weigh each meal to assure the meals all weigh the same, within a few tenths of an ounce.

Dinner - 4 Blocks

	Stuffed Orange Roughy for 3	P	C	F
12 oz.	Orange Roughy (or any other white fish)	64.0	0	4.0
-	Fat Free Cooking Spray	0	0	0
2 T	Butter	0	0	22.0
1 T	Lemon juice	0	1.0	0
-	Salt & Pepper to taste	0	0	0
Rice Stuffing:				
1 C	White Rice, cooked	4.0	38.0	0
½ C	Carrots, diced small	1.0	11.5	0
½ C	Peas, frozen	3.7	6.0	0.2
2 T	Green Onion tops, sliced	0.2	0.6	0
4	Lemon Slices, thin sliced	0	1.0	0
1 can	Asparagus	7.0	7.0	0
1 T	Butter	0	0	11.0
Mandarin Orange Salad:				
3 C	Romaine Lettuce	9.0	15.0	0
¼ C	Mandarin Oranges, light	0.5	8.0	0
15	Grapes	0	7.5	0
2 T	Mandarin Orange Salad Dressing	0	6.0	2.2
		89.4	101.6	39.4
		12.7	11.2	13.1
		4.2	3.7	4.3

Mandarin Orange Salad Dressing: Makes 4 Tablespoons.
1 t	Canola Oil
3 T	Mandarin Orange liquid, light
1 t	Red Wine Vinegar
1 t	Cider Vinegar
1 t	Sugar

Prepare rice as directed on package but omit the butter. About 5 minutes before the rice is done, add the diced carrots, peas and green onion tops. Continue cooking until vegetables are tender.

Thaw fish in milk. Discard the left over milk. Spray a cool skillet with fat free cooking spray and add 2 T butter. Heat skillet, sprinkle the fish with salt and pepper, squeeze the lemon juice evenly over fish, and fry fish until it flakes. (7 to 10 min) Heat asparagus and melt the butter over the top.

Divide rice stuffing and arrange on plate. When fish is done lay fish on top of rice stuffing and serve with a salad.

Combine salad dressing ingredients, shake well and pour 2 Tablespoons of dressing over the lettuce, mix well, divide and place in bowls. Cut grapes in half. Divide mandarin oranges and grapes and place on top of lettuce.

Divide and weigh each meal to assure the meals all weigh the same, within a few tenths of an ounce.

Dinner - 4 Blocks

Fillet of Sole for 3		P	C	F
16 oz.	Fillet of Sole	63.8	0	3.8
1½ T	Flour	1.2	8.2	0
-	Fat Free Cooking Spray	0	0	0
1 T	Butter	0	0	11.0
4 T	Heinz Ketchup	0	16.0	0
11 oz.	Corn (canned)	8.0	40.0	2.0
1 Can	Asparagus Spears	7.0	7.0	0
1½ T	Butter	0	0	16.5
Mandarin Orange Salad:				
4 C	Romaine Lettuce	12.0	20.0	0
¼ C	Mandarin Oranges, light	0.5	8.0	0
10	Grapes	0	5.0	0
3 T	Mandarin Orange Salad Dressing	0	9.0	3.3
		92.7	113.2	36.6
		13.2	12.5	12.2
		4.4	4.1	4.0

Mandarin Orange Salad Dressing: Makes 4 Tablespoons
- 1 t   Canola Oil
- 3 T   Mandarin Orange liquid, light
- 1 t   Red Wine Vinegar
- 1 t   Cider Vinegar
- 1 t   Sugar

Thaw frozen fish in milk, or if it's fresh, soak in the milk until ready to cook. Discard the left over milk. Spray a cool skillet with a fat free cooking spray; add 1 Tablespoons of butter and heat.

Season fish with salt and pepper and fry until fish flakes. Heat vegetables and melt 1½ Tablespoons of butter over the top.

Combine salad dressing ingredients, shake well and pour 3 Tablespoons of dressing over the lettuce, mix well, divide and place in bowls. Cut grapes in half. Divide mandarin oranges and grapes, place on top of lettuce.

(You can omit the grapes and mandarin oranges and still have a balanced meal.)

Divide and weigh each meal to assure the meals all weigh the same, within a few tenths of an ounce.

Dinner - 4 Blocks

Oriental Stir-Fry Shrimp for 3

		P	C	F
12 oz.	Shrimp, shelled	72.0	0	4.8
-	Fat Free Cooking Spray	0	0	0
2 T	Olive Oil	0	0	28.0
¼ C	Sherry, cooking	0	2.0	0
2 T	Soy Sauce	2.0	2.0	0
4 t	Corn Starch	0	9.2	0
½ t	Ginger, ground	0	0	0
½ C	Green Onions	1.0	2.5	0
¼ t	Garlic Powder	0	0	0
1 C	Broccoli	3.0	6.0	0.5
1 C	Cauliflower	2.0	5.0	0
¾ C	Snow Peas	3.0	9.0	0
½ C	Green Pepper	0.4	5.6	0
1½ C	White Rice, cooked	6.0	57.0	0
2 t	Sunflower Seeds	2.0	2.0	5.3
		91.4	100.3	38.6
		13.0	11.1	12.8
		4.3	3.7	4.2

Prepare rice as directed on package but omit the butter.

Stir together, cornstarch, sherry, soy sauce, ground ginger, salt, oregano, pepper and garlic. Add shrimp and coat well.

When ready to serve, cook rice according to directions on the box, but omit the butter. Spray a cool skillet with no-stick spray; add the oil and heat. Add the shrimp and stir-fry for about 3 minutes, or until shrimp are pink.

Remove the shrimp and add the vegetables. Stir-fry until the vegetables are crisp-tender. Return the shrimp to the skillet and heat just until hot. Divide the shrimp and rice by 3. Put shrimp mixture over rice and sprinkle with sunflower seeds.

Divide and weigh each meal to assure the meals all weigh the same, within a few tenths of an ounce.

Dinner - 4 Blocks

Grilled Orange Roughy and Apple Cole Slaw for 3

		P	C	F
12 oz.	Orange Roughy (or any other white fish)	63.7	0	3.9
-	Fat Free Cooking Spray	0	0	0
2½ T	Butter	0	0	27.5
1½ t	Lemon Juice	0	0.5	0
3 T	Miracle Whip, fat free	0	6.0	0
1 T	Sweet Pickle Relish	0.1	5.3	0.1
2 C	Cabbage, shredded	2.0	8.0	0
½	Apple, medium chopped	0	8.7	0
2 T	Raisins, dark	0.7	15.2	0
1	Celery Stalk, chopped	0	2.0	0
3 T	Miracle Whip, fat free	0	6.0	0
½ T	Milk 2%	0	0	0
½ T	Cider Vinegar	0	0.4	0
1 Can	Asparagus	7.0	7.0	0
11 oz.	Corn (canned)	8.0	40.0	2.0
		81.5	99.1	33.5
		11.6	11.0	11.1
		3.8	3.6	3.7

Grate cabbage and put in a large bowl. Chop apples and celery. Place in a bowl. Mix the dressing, pour over the slaw and set aside.

Mix miracle whip and sweet pickle relish and set aside. (You can omit the 3 Tablespoons of Miracle Whip and the sweet pickle relish and add 3 Tablespoons of Ketchup and still be in balance.)

Thaw frozen fish in milk, or if it's fresh, soak in the milk until ready to cook. Discard the left over milk. Spray a cool skillet with a fat free cooking spray and add 1½ t of butter. Heat skillet; sprinkle the fish with salt and pepper. Fry fish until the fish flakes. (7 to 10 minutes.)

Heat vegetables, divide the remaining 1 tablespoon of butter and melt over top. When ready to serve the apple Cole slaw divide the raisins and sprinkle on top of each bowl.

Divide and weigh each meal to assure the meals all weigh the same, within a few tenths of an ounce.

Dinner - 4 Blocks

Cheesy Fish Fillets for 3

		P	C	F
10.5 oz.	Fillet of Sole	55.8	0	3.0
1 T	Flour	0.7	5.5	0
½ T	Butter	0	0	7.3
-	Fat Free Cooking Spray	0	0	0
¾ oz.	Gruyere Cheese, grated	6.3	0	6.8
¾ oz.	Monterey Jack Cheese, light, grated	6.7	0.2	4.5
1 C	Milk 2%	8.0	12.0	5.0
2 T	Green Onion tops	0	0	0
1½ C	Broccoli	4.5	9.0	0.7
1½ C	Cauliflower	3.0	7.5	0
1 T	Butter	0	0	11.0
3 slices	Wheat Bread, Pepperidge Farm, light	7.0	22.0	1.0
Dessert:				
3 C	Peaches, fresh (2½" each)	0	27.0	0
1 C	Cool Whip, fat free	0	24.0	0
1 t	Sugar	0	4.0	0
		92.0	111.2	39.3
		13.1	12.3	13.1
		4.3	4.1	4.3

Thaw frozen fish in milk, or if it's fresh, soak in the milk until ready to cook. Discard the left over milk. Spray a cool skillet with a fat free cooking spray. Heat skillet. Coat the fish with flour and fry until it flakes easily.

Melt cheese and whisk with milk until smooth, and stir in the green onions. When fish is done, place on the plates, and cover with the cheese sauce.

Steam vegetables and melt the butter over the top. Serve fresh peaches and cool whip for dessert.

(You can substitute 2 medium Apples, or 2 Cups of Fruit Cocktail, water packed, for the peaches, cool whip and sugar. Or try another substitution.)

Divide and weigh each meal to assure the meals all weigh the same, within a few tenths of an ounce.

Dinner - 4 Blocks

Orange Roughy for 3   P   C   F

10.5 oz.	Orange Roughy (or any other white fish)	55.9	0	3.5
3 T	Parmesan Cheese, fat free	4.5	13.5	0
-	Fat Free Cooking Spray	0	0	0
1 C	Brussels Sprouts	6.0	20.0	1.0
½ C	Carrots, sliced	1.0	11.5	0
2 T	Butter	0	0	22.0
4 C	Romaine Lettuce	12.0	20.0	0
¼ C	Mandarin Oranges, light	0.5	8.0	0
1 T	Sunflower seeds	3.0	3.0	8.0
3 T	Mandarin Orange Salad Dressing	0	0.6	3.4
4 T	Heinz Ketchup **or**	0	16.0	0
8 T	Miracle Whip, regular	0	16.0	0
		82.9	108.9	37.9
		11.8	12.0	12.6
		3.9	4.0	4.2

Mandarin Orange Salad Dressing: Makes 4 Tablespoons.

1 t	Canola Oil
3 T	Mandarin Orange liquid, light
1 t	Red Wine Vinegar
1 t	Cider Vinegar
1 t	Sugar

Thaw frozen fish in milk, or if it's fresh, soak in the milk until ready to cook. Discard the left over milk.

Spray skillet with fat free cooking spray and heat. Sprinkle salt and pepper and Parmesan Cheese over fish and fry, turning once, until fish flakes.

Steam vegetables and melt the butter the top. Serve with salad.

Tear up lettuce and place in a bowl. Shake salad dressing well, pour 3 T of dressing over the lettuce and blend well. Divide lettuce equally into 3 salad bowls. Divide mandarin oranges and place on top of lettuce. Sprinkle 1 t of the sunflower seed on top of each salad.

Divide and weigh each meal to assure the meals all weigh the same, within a few tenths of an ounce.

Dinner - 4 Blocks

Marinated Shrimp in Almond Sauce for 3		P	C	F
12 oz.	Shrimp, large, (about 12 each)	72.0	0	4.8
1 T	Flour	0	5.0	0
-	Fat Free Cooking Spray	0	0	0
½ C	White Wine	0	0	0
1 t	Butter	0	0	3.6
1½ C	Mushrooms, fresh, sliced	3.0	6.0	0
½ C	Onion, thinly sliced	0.9	5.6	0.1
2	Cloves Garlic, minced	0	0	0
½ C	Tomato, seeded and chopped	0	3.0	0
8 oz.	Clam Juice	1.0	0	0
½ t	Thyme, dried, crushed	0	0	0
¼ t	Cinnamon	0	0	0
1	Bay Leaf	0	0	0
2 T	Almonds, ground	6.0	6.0	16.0
1 C	Snow Peas	4.0	12.0	0
1 T	Butter	0	0	11.0
2 oz.	Angel Hair Spaghetti	6.6	53.2	1.2
1 C	Lettuce, leafy	3.0	5.0	0
1 C	Strawberries	1.0	7.0	0
15	Grapes	0	7.5	0
1 T	Mandarin Orange Salad Dressing	0	3.0	1.1
		97.5	113.3	37.8
		13.9	12.5	12.6
		4.6	4.1	4.2

Mandarin Orange Salad Dressing: Makes 4 Tablespoons.
- 1 t — Canola Oil
- 3 T — Mandarin Orange liquid, light
- 1 t — Red Wine Vinegar
- 1 t — Cider Vinegar
- 1 t — Sugar

Rinse shrimp and marinate in wine for 30 minutes. Toss shrimp with flour and set aside. Reserve wine. Spray a cool skillet with a fat free cooking spray, add the mushrooms and cook, stirring over medium heat until tender. (3 to 5 min.) Remove mushrooms to a bowl and keep warm.

Add shrimp to the skillet, cook, stirring, until shrimp turns opaque. (3 to 5 min.) Transfer shrimp to mushroom bowl. Add the butter to the skillet and cook onion and garlic until tender. Stir in chopped tomato and reserved wine. Bring wine mixture to a boil; add the clam juice, thyme, cinnamon and bay leaf. Bring to a boil; reduce heat and cook, uncovered for 10 minutes, stirring occasionally. Grind the almonds. Return mushrooms and shrimp to the skillet. Add the almonds and heat just until shrimp and mushrooms are warm. Remove bay leaf; add salt and pepper to taste. Serve with salad and snow peas.

Divide and weigh each meal to assure the meals all weigh the same, within a few tenths of an ounce.

Pork Dinner Choices

Dinner - 4 Blocks

Baked Pork Loin Chops with Sweet Potatoes for 3

		P	C	F
12 oz	Pork Loin Chops	68.0	0	20.0
-	Fat Free Cooking Spray	0	0	0
1 T	Butter	0	0	11.0
½ C	Orange Juice	2.0	26.0	0
1 T	Brown sugar	0	12.0	0
¼ t	Ground Ginger	0	0	0
-	Salt and Pepper to taste	0	0	0
2	Sweet Potatoes	4.4	29.7	0.8
1 T	Butter	0	0	11.0
2 t	Cornstarch	0	4.6	0
1 can	Peas	14.0	24.5	1.7
¼ C	Rice, raw (1 Cup cooked)	4.0	38.0	0
		92.4	134.8	44.5
		13.2	14.9	14.8
		4.4	4.9	4.9

Make rice according to directions on the box.

Spray a cool skillet with fat free cooking spray; add the butter and brown the pork chops. Place in a baking pan. In a saucepan, combine orange juice, brown sugar, ginger, salt and pepper. Bring to a boil. Pour over the chops, cover and bake at 350 degrees for 30 minutes. Peel the sweet potatoes and cut into slices. Melt the butter and coat the potatoes.

Turn the chops over and cover with sweet potatoes, baste with the pan juices, cover and bake another 30 minutes, or until potatoes are tender.

About 20 minutes before sweet potatoes are done, cook the rice. When chops are done, remove along with the potatoes and cover to keep warm. Dissolve cornstarch in water and stir into the pan drippings. Bring to a boil, stirring, about 2 minutes.

Divide rice and put on plates. Place a pork loin chop and sweet potatoes over rice on each plate and pour pan juices over the top. Heat the peas and serve.

Divide and weigh each meal to assure the meals all weigh the same, within a few tenths of an ounce.

Dinner - 4 Blocks

Boneless B.B.Q. Pork"Ribs" for 3

		P	C	F
12 oz.	Pork Loin, boneless	68.0	0	20.0
¾ C	Open Pit Original B.B.Q. Sauce	0	22.0	0
11 oz.	Corn (canned)	8.0	40.0	2.0
1 can	Asparagus Spears	7.0	7.0	0
1½ T	Butter	0	0	16.5
		83.0	113.0	38.5
		11.8	12.5	12.8
		3.9	4.1	4.2

* You will actually only use about ¼ C of the Barbecue Sauce.

Trim all visible fat from the boneless pork loin, weigh and slice it in horizontally in half. Cut each half crosswise into strips. Toss "ribs" in barbecue sauce to coat and let stand, covered until ready to grill.

Place "ribs" in a 2 quart Dutch oven, heat over high heat until it boils. Turn the heat down to low and simmer until the "ribs" are almost tender. Remove to a platter.

Heat grill. Add ribs to grill and cook until they are lightly browned on the outside and just lose their pink in the center. (About 5 minutes, turning once.)

Heat corn and asparagus. Remove to serving bowls, divide the butter in half and melt over heated vegetables.

Divide and weigh each meal to assure the meals all weigh the same, within a few tenths of an ounce.

Dinner - 4 Blocks

	Pork Loin Chops with Cole Slaw for 3	P	C	F
10.5 oz.	Pork Loin Chops (3.5 oz. each)	65.1	0	21.0
-	Fat Free Cooking Spray	0	0	0
-	Salt and Pepper to taste	0	0	0
1 can	Asparagus Spears	7.0	7.0	0
1½ C	Cauliflower	3.0	7.5	0
1 can	Beets	3.0	21.0	0
1½ T	Butter	0	0	16.5
Cole Slaw:				
2 C	Cabbage, shredded	2.0	6.6	0
4 T	Miracle Whip, fat free	0	8.0	0
1 T	Milk 2%	0.5	0.7	0.3
1 t	Cider Vinegar	0	0	0
2 t	Sugar	0	8.0	0
1 can	Fruit Cocktail, in juice	0	49.0	0
		80.6	107.8	37.8
		11.5	11.9	12.6
		3.8	3.9	4.2

Mix together, miracle whip, milk, cider vinegar and sugar. Shred cabbage. Pour mixture over shredded cabbage and chill.

Trim all visible fat from the pork chops. (Remove fat before weighing) Spray a cool skillet with a fat free cooking spray and heat. Fry pork chops until the meat is no longer pink.

Heat the beets and asparagus. Steam the cauliflower. Melt ½ Tablespoon of the butter over each vegetable.

Divide the fruit cocktail and have for dessert. (You can omit the fruit cocktail and add 5 Cups of diced watermelon and still be in balance. Or try another substitution.)

Divide and weigh each meal to assure the meals all weigh the same, within a few tenths of an ounce.

Dinner - 4 Blocks

Pork Chops with Stuffing and for 3		P	C	F
12 oz.	Pork Chops	68.0	0	20.0
-	Fat Free Cooking Spray	0	0	0
2 C	Chicken Stuffing Mix	12.0	76.0	1.2
1 can	Asparagus	7.0	7.0	0
1½ T	Butter	0	0	16.5
2 C	Romaine Lettuce	6.0	10.0	0
¼ C	Mandarin Oranges, light	0.5	8.0	0
10	Grapes	0	5.0	0
1 C	Strawberries, sliced	1.0	7.0	0
2 T	Mandarin Orange Salad Dressing	0	6.0	2.2
		94.5	119.0	39.9
		13.5	13.2	13.3
		4.5	4.4	4.4

Mandarin Orange Salad Dressing: Makes 4 Tablespoons.
- 1 t   Canola Oil
- 3 T   Mandarin Orange liquid, light
- 1 t   Red Wine Vinegar
- 1 t   Cider Vinegar
- 1 t   Sugar

(Remove all visible fat from the pork chops before weighing.)

Spray a cool skillet with a fat free cooking spray and fry pork chops until they are no longer pink. Make the Stove Top Stuffing, but omit the butter and substitute the 4 tablespoons of chicken broth. Use only 2 cups of the stuffing. Heat the asparagus and melt the butter over it.

(You can omit the asparagus, use 1½ Cups of dressing and an 11-oz. can of corn, and the meal will still be balanced.)

Combine salad dressing ingredients, shake well and pour 2 Tablespoons of dressing over the lettuce, mix well, divide and place in bowls. Cut grapes in half. Chop strawberries. Divide mandarin oranges grapes and strawberries and place on top of lettuce.

(You can omit the grapes or strawberries and still have a balanced meal.)

Divide and weigh each meal to assure the meals all weigh the same, within a few tenths of an ounce.

Dinner - 4 Blocks

Pork Teriyaki with Mandarin Orange Salad for 3

		P	C	F
12 oz.	Pork Teriyaki Tenderloin	63.0	12.0	12.0
½ C	Carrots, diced	1.0	11.5	0
2 C	Cauliflower	4.0	10.0	0
1½ C	Brussels Sprouts	12.0	40.0	2.6
4 t	Butter	0	0	12.8

Mandarin Orange Salad:

		P	C	F
3 C	Romaine Lettuce	9.0	15.0	0
¼ C	Mandarin Oranges, light	0.5	8.0	0
10	Grapes	0	5.0	0
1 C	Strawberries, sliced	1.0	7.0	0
1 T	Almonds, slivered	3.0	3.0	8.0
2 T	Mandarin Orange Salad Dressing	0	6.0	2.2
		93.5	117.5	37.6
		13.3	13.0	12.5
		4.4	4.3	4.1

Mandarin Orange Salad Dressing: Makes 4 Tablespoons.

1 t	Canola Oil
3 T	Mandarin Orange liquid, light
1 t	Red Wine Vinegar
1 t	Cider Vinegar
1 t	Sugar

Purchase a Teriyaki Pork Tenderloin and cut it into 12 oz. pieces. (One package usually serves about 3 meals.) Slice the 12 ounces into about 1½" thick slices. (Or buy regular Pork Tenderloin and use my Teriyaki Marinade recipe on page 260.

Grill pork until no longer pink. Steam vegetables, melt the butter over them and divide by 3.

Make the salad dressing, shake well and pour 3 Tablespoons over the lettuce, mix well, divide and place in the bowls. Cut up the grapes and strawberries. Divide and place on top of lettuce. Divide the mandarin oranges and place on top of lettuce. Put 1 Teaspoon of slivered almonds on each salad.

(You can omit the grapes and strawberries and still have a balanced meal.)

Divide and weigh each meal to assure the meals all weigh the same, within a few tenths of an ounce.

Dinner -5 Blocks

Pork Teriyaki with Chocolate Mousse for 3

		P	C	F
14 oz.	Pork Teriyaki Tenderloin	73.5	14.0	14.0
½ C	Carrots, diced	1.0	11.5	0
2 C	Cauliflower	4.0	10.0	0
1½ C	Brussels Sprouts	12.0	40.0	2.6
1½ T	Butter	0	0	16.5
2/3 C	Milk, 2%	4.0	5.5	3.3
¾ pkg.	Chocolate Mousse Mix	12.0	40.0	10.0
1½ C	Strawberries	1.5	10.5	0
2 t	Sugar	0	8.0	0
		108.0	139.5	46.4
		15.4	15.5	15.4
		5.1	5.1	5.1

Make Chocolate Mousse and chill until dinner.

Purchase a Teriyaki Pork Tenderloin, remove all visible fat and cut it into 12 oz. pieces. (Weigh the pork teriyaki after the fat has been removed.) (One package usually serves about 3 meals.)

Slice the 12 ounces into about 1½" thick slices. Or buy regular Pork Tenderloin and use my Teriyaki Marinade recipe on page 260.

Grill pork until no longer pink. Steam vegetables, melt the butter over them and divide by 3.

Slice strawberries and stir in sugar.

Divide and weigh each meal to assure the meals all weigh the same, within a few tenths of an ounce.

Dinner - 5 Blocks

		P	C	F
Pork Roast and Vegetables for 3				
12 oz.	Pork Tenderloin	68.0	0	20.0
-	Fat Free Cooking Spray	0	0	0
1½ T	Butter	0	0	16.5
1 C	Onions, diced	1.8	11.2	0.2
6	Potatoes, New Red small (12 oz.)	3.9	27.9	0
1½ C	Carrots diced (5.5 oz.)	2.0	23.0	0
Mandarin Orange Salad:				
1 C	Romaine Lettuce	3.0	5.0	0
¼ C	Mandarin Oranges, light	0.5	8.0	0
10	Grapes	0	5.0	0
1 C	Strawberries, sliced	1.0	7.0	0
1 T	Mandarin Orange Salad Dressing	0	3.0	1.1
12 oz.	Milk, 2% (4 oz. each)	12.0	16.5	7.5
3 slices	Wheat Bread, Pepperidge Farm, light	7.0	22.0	1.0
		99.2	128.6	46.3
		14.1	14.2	15.4
		4.7	4.7	5.1

Mandarin Orange Salad Dressing: Makes 4 Tablespoons

1 t	Canola Oil
3 T	Mandarin Orange liquid, light
1 t	Red Wine Vinegar
1 t	Cider Vinegar
1 t	Sugar

Spray an electric skillet with a fat free cooking spray and add 1½ Tablespoons of butter. Trim as much visible fat from the pork roast as possible. Sprinkle meat lightly with salt and pepper. Brown the pork roast on all sides. Add about ½ cup of water, and cover. Cook for about 30 minutes, or until the meat is pale pink.

Cut the onion into about 8 pieces. Peel potatoes and carrots and cut into bite size pieces. Add the onions, potatoes, and carrots. Put potatoes on one side of the pork and the carrots on the other side. (It's easier to divide when you are ready to serve.) Cook until the vegetables are tender and the pork roast is no longer pink. Serve one slice of bread per serving. **Don't put any butter on the bread.**

Combine salad dressing ingredients, shake well and pour 1 Tablespoon of dressing over the lettuce, mix well, divide and place in bowls. Divide mandarin oranges, strawberries, and grapes, place on top of lettuce.

(You can omit the grapes and/or strawberries and still have a balanced meal.)
Divide and weigh each meal to assure the meals all weigh the same, within a few tenths of an ounce.

Vegetarian Dinner Choices

Dinner - 4 Blocks

Eggplant Parmigiana for 4

		P	C	F
1	Eggplant (about 16 oz.)	4.7	16.3	0.8
-	Fat Free Cooking Spray	0	0	0
½ T	Butter	0	0	5.5
¼ C	Bread Crumbs, plain	4.0	18.0	1.5
1 T	Parmesan Cheese	0	0	0
2 T	Flour	1.5	10.0	0
2	Egg Whites, lightly beaten	8.0	0	0
1 t	Oregano	0	0	0
1 C	Marinara Sauce	8.0	18.0	10.0
3 oz.	Mozzarella Cheese, grated, reduced fat	27.0	3.0	6.0
		53.2	65.3	23.8
		7.6	7.2	7.9
		3.8	3.6	3.9

Preheat the oven to 350 degrees. Spray an 8x8x2-baking pan with a fat free cooking spray, add the ½ T butter and set aside.

Trim the ends from the eggplant. If desired, remove the skin. Slice the eggplant crosswise into ½ inch thick slices. Set aside.

Stir together the bread crumbs, Parmesan cheese and oregano. Dip the eggplant slices into the flour, then dip into the egg white and coat them with the bread crumb mixture.

Arrange the eggplant into the prepared pan. Bake for 20 to 25 minutes or until lightly brown. Remove from the oven.

Spoon the Marinara sauce over the eggplant. Sprinkle with the mozzarella cheese. Bake about 10 minutes more or until the cheese is melted.

Divide and weigh each meal to assure the meals all weigh the same, within a few tenths of an ounce.

Dinner 4- Blocks

Spicy Vegetarian Lasagna for 6

		P	C	F
6 oz	Tofu, extra firm	12.0	3.0	7.5
3 ½ T	Olive Oil	0	0	35.0
½ C	Onions, chopped	0.9	5.6	0.1
½ C	Green Peppers, chopped	0.4	5.6	0.1
1	Garlic Clove, crushed	0	0	0
2 cans	Black Beans	42.0	91.0	0
2 cans	Tomato Sauce (30 oz)	14.0	28.0	0
¼ C	Cilantro, fresh, chopped	0.1	0.1	0.1
2 C	Cottage Cheese, 2%	56.0	16.0	8.0
4 T	Sour Cream	1.2	2.0	10.0
6	Lasagna Noodles	16.8	96.0	2.4
9 T	Parmesan Cheese, grated	27.0	0	7.7
		170.4	244.3	70.9
		24.3	27.1	23.6
		4.0	4.5	3.9

Sauce:
Cook noodles according to the directions on the pan.

While they are cooking, put oil in a cool skillet and fry the tofu. Using a fork, crush the tofu while cooking until it's brown and crumbly. Add the onion, red bell pepper and garlic. Cook until tender.

Mash 1 can of black beans. Stir the mashed beans, along with the other can of beans, the tomato sauce and cilantro into the vegetables. Heat through.

Combine the cottage cheese and sour cream. Rinse the noodles with cold water and drain.

Spray a baking dish with fat free cooking spray. Arrange 3 noodles on the bottom. Top with 1/2 the vegetable sauce and cheese mixture. Put another layer of noodles and vegetable sauce with the cheese mixture. Bake, covered, in a 350-degree oven for 20 to 30 minutes, or until heated through.

Let stand about 10 minutes.

Divide and weigh each meal to assure the meals all weigh the same, within a few tenths of an ounce.

Dinner 4- Blocks

Vegetarian Chili for 3		P	C	F
16 oz	Tofu, extra firm	48.0	4.0	24.0
-	Fat Free Cooking Spray	0	0	0
1 T	Canola Oil	0	0	14.0
1 C	Green Pepper, chopped	0.8	11.2	0.2
1 C	Onions, chopped	1.8	11.2	0.2
1 C	Zucchini	2.0	4.0	0
14.5 oz	Whole tomatoes, canned	3.5	10.5	0
15 oz	Tomato Sauce	7.0	14.0	0
15 oz	Kidney Beans	24.5	52.5	1.0
¼ t	Red Pepper Flakes, crushed	0	0	0
3 slices	Wheat Bread, Pepperidge Farm, light	6.0	24.0	1.0
		97.1	131.4	40.4
		13.8	14.6	13.4
		4.6	4.8	4.4

Spray a cool skillet with Fat Free Cooking Spray; add the olive oil and heat. Crumble the tofu and stir until browned.

Add the next 6 ingredients, and the red pepper flakes if you like it a little hot, and simmer for about an hour.

Divide and weigh each meal to assure the meals all weigh the same, within a few tenths of an ounce.

Dinner 4- Blocks

Vegetarian Fried Rice for 3		P	C	F
16 oz	Tofu, extra Firm	48.0	4.0	24.0
½ T	Olive Oil	0	0	7.0
1	Egg, Whole	6.0	0	5.0
4	Egg Whites	16.0	0	0
1 ½ C	Onions, chopped	2.7	16.8	0.3
1 pkg.	Fried Rice Seasoning Mix	3.0	18.0	0
½ C	White Rice, raw (2 Cups Cooked)	8.0	76.0	0
	Salt and Pepper to taste	0	0	0
		83.7	114.8	36.3
		11.9	12.7	12.1
		4.0	4.2	4.0

Cook rice according to package but don't use any butter.

Spray a cool skillet with fat free cooking spray; add the olive oil and scramble the tofu and onions with the Fried Rice Seasoning Mix until brown.

Whisk the egg and egg whites together and scramble with the tofu mixture.

Add the cooked rice and stir until blended well.

2 Block Snack Choices

2 Block Snacks

		P	C	F
5	Waverly Crackers	1.0	10.0	3.5
11	Pizza Style Canadian bacon	4.5	0	2.0
1 oz.	Cheddar Cheese, fat free	8.0	1.0	0
1	Sweet Pickle, medium	0	8.0	0
		13.5	19.0	5.5
		1.9	2.1	1.8

		P	C	F
6	Anchovies, oil packed	4.0	0	1.5
5	Waverly Crackers	1.0	10.0	3.5
1 oz.	Cheddar Cheese, fat free	8.0	1.0	0
1	Sweet Pickle, medium	0	8.0	0
		13.5	19.0	5.5
		1.9	2.1	1.8

		P	C	F
2 oz.	Tuna, Albacore, water pack	15.0	0	1.0
2 T	Green Onions, chopped	0.2	0.6	0
2 T	Miracle Whip, fat free	0	4.0	0
8	Waverly Crackers	1.6	16.0	5.6
		16.8	20.6	6.6
		2.4	2.2	2.2

		P	C	F
¼ C	Cocktail Sauce	1.0	12.0	0.5
9	Shrimp, large	15.0	0	1.0
1 t	Lemon Juice	0	0.3	0
5	Green Olives, medium	0	0	3.0
		16.0	12.3	4.5
		2.2	1.4	1.5

Sour Cream and Onion Dip

		P	C	F
3 oz.	Sour Cream, regular Onion Dip Mix	1.2	6.0	7.5
15	Pringles Fat Free Chips	1.7	15.0	0
1.5 oz.	Cheddar Cheese, fat free	12.0	1.5	0
		14.9	22.5	7.5
		2.1	2.5	2.5

2 Block Snacks

Chicken Chimichangas (12 - 2 block snack)

		P	C	F
16.8 oz.	Chicken Breasts, skinless, boneless	109.2	0	6.7
16 oz.	Pace Salsa	0	42.0	0
1 t	Butter	0	0	3.6
1½ C	Refried Beans, fat free (1 can)	21.0	36.0	0
12	Manny's Flour Tortillas, 6"	12.0	144.0	12.0
1 T	Taco Seasoning	0	4.5	0
8 oz.	Cheddar Cheese, regular, grated	56.0	8.0	72.0
8 oz.	Green Chili's, diced	1.0	8.0	0
		199.2	242.5	94.3
		28.4	26.9	31.4
		2.3	2.2	2.6

Remove skin and all visible fat from the chicken. Boil the chicken breasts until done. Shred the cooked chicken breasts with a fork. Place the shredded chicken into a large bowl, add salsa, refried beans, taco seasoning, green chili's, melted butter and grated cheese. Stir until well blended.

Divide the meat mixture into 12 equal portions and place in the center of the flour tortillas. Roll the tortillas. The Chicken mixture should weigh about 70.0 ounces, making about 4.5 ounces of chicken mixture for each tortilla. Chimichangas should weigh from 5.0 to 5.5 ounces including the 6" tortilla. Place in plastic bags and freeze until ready to eat. When ready to eat, thaw chimi and then heat in a conventional oven or a toaster oven only until hot. (If you are in a hurry you can microwave the chimi but the tortilla will be a little rubbery)

Shredded Beef Chimichangas (12-2 Block Snacks)

		P	C	F
16 oz.	Top Round Roast, lean	122.8	0	17.2
-	Fat Free Cooking Spray	0	0	0
1	Beef Bouillon Cube	0	1.0	0
16 oz.	Pace Salsa	0	42.0	0
1½ C	Refried Beans, fat free (1 can)	21.0	36.0	0
12	Manny's Flour Tortillas (6")	12.0	144.0	12.0
1 T	Taco Seasoning	0	4.5	0
8 oz.	Cheddar Cheese, regular, grated	56.0	8.0	72.0
8 oz.	Green Chiles, diced	1.0	8.0	0
		212.8	243.5	101.2
		30.4	27.0	33.7
		2.5	2.2	2.8

You can substitute 93% lean hamburger for the top round roast, add all the rest of the ingredients, (skip the cooking spray and bouillon cube) and make ground beef chimichangas.

Remove all visible fat from the beef. Spray a cool skillet with non-stick spray; add the beef and brown. When the beef is brown, add some water and the bouillon cube cover and boil until the beef is fork tender. Let the meat cool and then shred with a fork. Place the shredded beef into a large bowl; add salsa, refried beans, taco seasoning, green chiles and grated cheese. Stir until well blended.

Divide the meat mixture into 12 equal portions and place in the center of the flour tortillas. Roll the tortillas. The Beef mixture should weigh about 70.0 ounces, making about 4.5 to 5 ounces of beef mixture for each tortilla. Chimichangas should weigh from 5.5 to 6.0 ounces including the 6" tortilla. Place in plastic bags and freeze until ready to eat. When ready to eat, thaw chimi and then heat in a conventional oven or a toaster oven only until hot. (If you are in a hurry you can microwave the chimi but the tortilla will be a little rubbery.)

2 Block Snacks

Shredded B.B.Q. Pork Tenderloin Chimi's (12-2 Block Snacks)

		P	C	F
16 oz.	Pork Tenderloin, trimmed, boneless	95.2	0	15.5
16 oz.	Pace Salsa	0	42.0	0
¼ C	Open Pit B.B.Q. Sauce, original	0	22.0	0
1½ C	Refried Beans, fat free (1 can)	21.0	36.0	0
12	Manny's Flour Tortillas, 6"	12.0	144.0	12.0
1 T	Taco Seasoning	0	4.5	0
8 oz.	Cheddar Cheese, regular, grated	56.0	8.0	72.0
8 oz.	Green Chili's, diced	1.0	8.0	0
		185.2	264.5	99.5
		26.4	29.3	33.1
		2.2	2.4	2.7

Remove all visible fat from the pork tenderloin. Marinate Pork Tenderloin in the B.B.Q. sauce for 2 hours. Place marinated pork into a roast pan and roast until the pork is no longer pink, the juices run clear and is fork tender. Let cool. Shred the pork with a fork and place in a large bowl. Add salsa, refried beans, taco seasoning, green chili's, and grated cheese. Stir until well blended.

Divide the meat mixture into 12 equal portions and place in the center of the flour tortillas. Roll the tortillas. The pork mixture should weigh about 70.0 ounces, making about 4.5 ounces of chicken mixture for each tortilla. Chimichangas should weigh from 5.0 to 5.5 ounces including the 6" tortilla. Place in plastic bags and freeze until ready to eat. When ready to eat, thaw chimi and then heat in a conventional oven or a toaster oven only until hot. (If you are in a hurry you can microwave the chimi but the tortilla will be a little rubbery)

Grilled Ham and Cheese Sandwich

		P	C	F
2 slices	Wheat Bread, Pepperidge Farm, light	4.0	14.0	0.5
2 slices	American Cheese, reduced fat	8.0	4.0	6.0
½ T	Miracle Whip, fat free	0	1.0	0
1 slice	Cooked Ham, 96% extra lean	5.0	0	1.0
4	Pringles Fat Free Potato Chips	0.5	4.0	0
-	Salt and Pepper to taste	0	0	0
		17.5	23.0	7.5
		2.5	2.5	2.5

		P	C	F
½ C	Cottage Cheese 2%	14.0	4.0	2.0
1 C	Peach, fresh, sliced	1.2	16.2	0
½ T	Almonds, slivered	1.5	1.5	4.0
		16.7	21.7	6.0
		2.3	2.4	2.0

2 Block Snacks

		P	F	C
½ C	Cottage Cheese 2%	14.0	4.0	2.0
½ C	Peach slices, canned, in juice	0	14.0	0
½ T	Almonds, slivered	1.5	1.5	4.0
		15.5	19.5	6.0
		2.2	2.2	2.0

		P	C	F
½ C	Cottage Cheese 2%	14.0	4.0	2.0
½ C	Pineapple, crush, light	0.5	16.0	0.5
½ T	Almonds, slivered	2.0	2.0	4.0
		16.5	22.0	6.5
		2.3	2.4	2.1

		P	C	F
½ C	Cottage Cheese 2%	14.0	4.0	2.0
½ C	Mandarin Oranges, light	1.0	16.0	0
½ T	Almonds, slivered	2.0	2.0	4.0
		17.0	22.0	6.0
		2.4	2.4	2.0

		P	C	F
½ C	Cottage Cheese 2%	14.0	4.0	2.0
½ C	Fruit Cocktail, light	0	14.0	0
½ T	Almonds, slivered	1.5	1.5	4.0
		15.5	19.5	6.0
		2.2	2.2	2.0

		P	C	F
½ C	Cottage Cheese 2%	14.0	4.0	2.0
2 C	Strawberries	2.0	14.0	0
½ T	Almonds, slivered	1.5	1.5	4.0
		17.5	19.5	6.0
		2.5	2.2	2.0

		P	C	F
½ C	Cottage Cheese 2%	14.0	4.0	2.0
1 C	Blackberries	1.0	11.2	0
½ T	Almonds, slivered	1.5	1.5	4.0
		16.5	16.7	6.0
		2.3	1.9	2.0

2 Block Snacks

		P	C	F
½ C	Cottage Cheese 2%	14.0	4.0	2.0
1 C	Raspberries	1.0	14.0	0
½ T	Almonds, slivered	2.0	2.0	4.0
		17.0	20.0	6.0
		2.4	2.2	2.0

Hot Chocolate

		P	C	F
2 T	Chocolate Drink Mix, Sugar Free	1.0	5.0	1.0
8 oz.	Milk, 2%	8.0	11.0	5.0
		9.0	16.0	6.0
		1.3	1.7	2.0

		P	C	F
1	Nutritionally Balanced Bar	2.0	2.0	2.0

4 Block snack for 1
Or
2 Block snack for 2

Chicken Teriyaki Nuggets for 1
3-oz	Chicken Breasts, skinless, boneless
3 T	flour
-	Salt and Pepper to taste
2 t	Oil

Teriyaki Marinade:
¼ C	Light Brown Sugar, packed
¼ C	Soy Sauce
2 T	Lemon Juice
1 T	Canola Oil
¼ t	Ground Ginger
1	Garlic Clove, minced

Cut chicken in 2-inch squares. Mix marinade ingredients and marinate the chicken for 3 hours. When ready to serve, combine flour, salt, and pepper. Coat chicken with seasoned flour. Spray a cool skillet with a fat free cooking spray, add oil and heat. Add chicken and cook, turning as needed until golden brown. Remove chicken from skillet. Serves 1.

Holiday Meals Section

Thanksgiving Turkey Dinner for 1
6 Blocks

Thanksgiving Turkey Dinner (Turkey Breast only)

		P	C	F
4 oz.	Turkey Breast, roasted, skinless	33.9	0	3.7
½ C	Traditional Sage Dressing	4.0	20.2	9.0
½ C	Potatoes, mashed	2.0	19.0	1.0
¼ C	Gravy	0.7	5.5	0.5
½	Deviled Egg	3.0	3.2	2.5
½ t	Butter	0	0	1.8
2	Sweet pickles, small	0	8.0	0
		43.6	55.9	18.5
		6.2	6.2	6.7

Thanksgiving Turkey Dinner (Dark Meat only)

		P	C	F
4 oz.	Turkey, Dark Meat, roasted, skinless	32.4	0	8.2
½ C	Traditional Sage Dressing	4.0	20.2	9.0
½ C	Potatoes, mashed	2.0	19.0	1.0
¼ C	Gravy	0.7	5.5	0.5
2	Sweet pickle, small	0	8.0	0
		39.1	52.7	18.7
		5.5	5.8	6.2

Stuff turkey just before roasting. Allow about ¾ C stuffing per pound ready to cook weight of turkey. Rinse bird and pat dry. Rub inside of cavities with salt, if desired. Spoon stuffing, loosely into wishbone cavity; skewer neck skin to back. Then, lightly spoon stuffing into large cavity. If opening has a band of skin across tail push the drumsticks under the band. If the band of skin is not present, tie legs together and then to the tail. Twist wing tips under back of turkey.

To roast: Place breast side up on a rack in a shallow roasting pan. Rub skin thoroughly with oil. If using a meat thermometer is used, insert into center of inside thigh muscle, not touching the bone. Cover turkey loosely with foil, pressing is lightly at drumsticks and breast ends. Avoid having foil touching top or sides. Roast in an uncovered pan according to directions on turkey wrap. (Depends on size of bird) When turkey is almost done, cut band of skin or string between legs and tail. Continue roasting until done.

Testing for doneness:

Check the turkey about 20 minutes before roasting time is up. The thickest part of the drumstick should feel soft when pressed between finger protected with a paper towel. Drumstick should move up and down and twist easily in the socket. Meat thermometer should register 185 degrees. Remove turkey from oven and let stand for 15 minutes before carving.

Deviled Eggs: Place eggs in cold water. Bring water to boil then turn off the heat. Cover and let the eggs stand in the water for 20 minutes. Remove from the pan and cover with cold water to loosen shell. Remove shell, cut egg in half, lengthwise, and remove the yolk. Mash the yolk and add the miracle whip, sugar and cider vinegar. Spoon mixture back into the eggs and sprinkle with a little paprika.

Serve with a pickle or a few tablespoons of cranberry sauce.

Christmas Ham Dinner For 3
7 Blocks

Double Smoked Ham
12 oz	Ham, double smoked, trim off fat
2 C	Potatoes, new red
4 oz	Cheddar Cheese, fat free
3 T	Butter
¼ C	Bread Crumbs
1½	Deviled Eggs
3	Sweet Pickles, small

7 Layer Salad:
2 C	Lettuce
½ C	Purple Onion, diced
2	Celery Stalks
½ C	Peas, canned
8 T	Miracle Whip, fat free
1 T	Sugar
3 slices	Bacon, lean
10 T	Parmesan Cheese, fat free

Dice the bacon and fry until crisp. Soak up the excess grease. Set aside. Chop up first 3 ingredients. Layer the vegetables, lettuce, celery and purple onion. Blend miracle whip and sugar together and pour over the salad mixture. Spread peas on top. Sprinkle Parmesan cheese over peas. Spread the bacon bits over cheese, and chill.

Peel potatoes, and place in a casserole dish, melt the butter and pour over the potatoes, add 2 oz. cheese, sprinkle on the bread crumbs and mix well. Heat oven to 350 degree and bake until the potatoes are almost done. Sprinkle the rest of the cheese on top and continue baking until potatoes are tender. Remove from oven and keep warm. Heat the ham according to directions on package. Can drink a glass of wine with dinner.

Thank Goodness Thanksgiving and Christmas only come once a year. As you know, it's never a good thing to eat more than 5 blocks for any one meal, but the holidays are special and I plan on enjoying my holiday dinners.

Of course, you can eat all you want for Thanksgiving and Christmas Dinners, this is just a menu in case you have the will power.

Personally, I plan on eating a balanced breakfast and lunch, a nice holiday dinner with all the trimmings, and then get back into balance with a 2 block snack about a half hour before going to bed.

Miscellaneous Choices

Honey Wheat Bread

		P	C	F
4 t	Yeast (2 pkgs.)	6.9	1.9	0.7
4 C	Lukewarm Water	0	0	0
2/3 C	Powdered Milk	16.0	24.0	0
1 T	Salt	0	0	0
¼ C	Honey	0	60.0	0
¼ C	Molasses	0	68.0	0
½ C	Brown Sugar	0	96.0	0
½ C	Canola Oil	0	0	112.0
5 C	Wheat Flour	80.0	360.0	0
5 C	White Flour	60.0	440.0	0
	5 Loaves = grams	162.9	1049.9	112.7
	1 Loaf = grams	23.2	116.6	37.5
	1 Loaf sliced into 18 slices = grams	1.2	6.4	2.0

1 slice of bread=1.2 grams of Protein
6.4 grams of Carbohydrates
2.0 grams of Fat

Heat oven to 350 degrees.

Dissolve the yeast in ½ C of lukewarm water. In mixer, mis3½ C water, salt, molasses, brown sugar, honey and oil. Add the wheat flour, powdered milk and dissolved yeast mixture and mix thoroughly. Let stand for 5 minutes. Add remaining flour, turn out on a floured surface and knead for 8 minutes. Place in a large greased bowl, turning to coat and cover with a damp towel. Let rise for 1 hour. Punch down, turn out on a floured surface and knead again until the dough is elastic. (About another 8 minutes.) Return to greased bowl and let rise until double. Punch down, shape into loaves and let rise until light. Bake in a 350-degree oven for about 30 minutes. The loaves will sound hollow when you tap on them. Makes 5 regular size loaves.

Bake for about 30 minutes. (Until loaf sounds hollow when you tap on it.)
Slice each loaf into 18 pieces.

Fruit Salad
This salad is not balanced alone; it must be eaten with a meal.

Apple-Cinnamon Fruit Salad for 3
3 C	Cabbage, shredded
½	Apple, chopped
10	Red Grapes, halved
3 T	Vanilla Yogurt
2 t	Milk 2%
-	Ground Cinnamon, dash
1 T	Sunflower Seeds

P	C	F
5.5	30.2	9.0

In a large bowl combine cabbage, chopped apple, and grapes.

Dressing:
In a small bowl, stir together yogurt, milk and cinnamon. Pour dressing over cabbage mixture. Toss lightly to coat. Cover and chill for 2 to 6 hours. Sprinkle with sunflower seeds just before serving.

Orange Salad for 3
This salad is not balanced alone; it must be eaten with a meal.

Orange Salad for 3
4 C	Mixed Greens, torn
½	Orange, medium, sectioned
½ C	Jicama, cut into thin strips
½	Red Onion, small, rings

Cranberry Vinaigrette Dressing:
2 T	Cranberry Juice Cocktail
½ T	Canola Oil
½ T	Vinegar
¼ t	Basil, dried, crushed
½ t	Sugar

P	C	F
13.7	39.0	7.1

In large bowl combine mixed greens, orange sections, jicama, and red onions. Shake Cranberry Juice Vinaigrette well and pour over salad. Toss lightly to coat. Serve immediately.

Salad Dressings
Marinades and Sauces

Mandarin Orange Salad Dressing: Makes 4 Tablespoons.
1 t	Canola Oil
3 T	Mandarin Orange liquid, light
1 t	Red Wine Vinegar
1 t	Cider Vinegar
1 t	Sugar

Cranberry Vinaigrette Dressing:
2 T	Cranberry Juice Cocktail
½ T	Canola Oil
½ T	Vinegar
¼ t	Basil, dried, crushed
½ t	Sugar

Tomato-Basil Vinaigrette dressing:
1	Tomato, medium
2 t	Canola Oil
1 T	Red Wine Vinegar
1 t	Dried Basil, crushed
1 t	Sugar
1/4 t	Horseradish
1/8 t	Pepper
1	Garlic clove, minced

Lemon Yogurt Dressing:
2 oz	Vanilla Yogurt Custard
1/2 t	Canola Oil
1/2 T	Miracle Whip, regular
½ t	Lemon Peel, finely shredded

Raspberry Dressing:
1/4 C	Raspberries
1 T	Sour Cream, fat free
2 T	Milk
1 t	Lemon Juice
1/8 t	Celery Seed

Raspberry Vinaigrette Dressing:
1 t	Raspberry Vinegar
¼ C	Raspberries
1 t	Sugar

Salad Dressings
Marinades and Sauces

Ginger Lime Marinade:
2 T	Lime Juice
2 T	Liquid from Mandarin Orange light can
1 t	Ginger Root
-	Salt to taste
-	Cayenne Pepper
1	Garlic, Clove

Herb Dressing:
4 T	Miracle Whip, fat free
2 T	Miracle Whip, regular
1/2 T	Lemon Juice
1/2 T	Dijon-style mustard
1/8 t	Black Pepper

Apricot Preserve Dressing:
3 T	Sour Cream, fat free
3 T	Apricot preserves
1 T	Red Wine Vinegar
1/2 T	Canola Oil
1/2 T	Miracle Whip, fat free
1/2 T	Soy Sauce
1/2 t	Prepared Mustard
1/8 t	Ground Cinnamon

Teriyaki Marinade:
¼ C	Light Brown Sugar, tightly packed
½ C	Soy Sauce
½ t	Monosodium Glutamate
¼ t	Pepper
2 T	Lemon Juice
1 T	Canola Oil
1 T	Ginger Root, grated / or 1 t dry ginger
2	Garlic Clove, minced

Mix together, add meat, stir to coat and marinate for 2 hours or refrigerate overnight.

Horseradish Cream Sauce:
1 C	Milk 2%
1 T	Cornstarch
2 T	Horseradish
1 t	Mustard, Grey Poupon
2	Whole Black Peppers
1	Garlic Clove, minced
1	Bay Leaf, crumbled
2 t	Worcestershire Sauce
½ t	Marjoram, dried

Salad Dressings
Marinades and Sauces

Lemon-Dill Mayonnaise:
4 T	Miracle Whip, fat free
½ T	Fresh Parsley, snipped
1 T	Fresh Dill, snipped
½ t	Lemon Zest
1 t	Lemon Juice
1	Garlic Clove, small, minced
2 T	Buttermilk

Hollandaise Sauce:
1	Egg Yolk
2 t	Lemon Juice
3 T	Water

White Sauce:
3 T	Water
1 T	Flour
½ C	Milk, 2%
¼ t	Salt
1/8 t	Paprika
-	Pepper

Marinara Sauce:
2 T	Olive Oil
2	Garlic Cloves
16 oz.	Whole Tomatoes
6 oz.	Tomato Paste
1 T	Sugar
2 t	Basil
1½ t	Salt

Balanced 3-Block Salads

Blocked Salads
This salad can be eaten alone as a 2-block meal.

Strawberry Salad for 1

3 T	Mandarin Orange Salad Dressing
1 t	Orange Peel, finely shredded
3 C	Mixed Greens
½ C	Strawberries, sliced
½ T	Pecans, chopped
1 T	Canola Oil
2 T	Mandarin Orange liquid, light
2 t	Red Wine Vinegar
1 t	Cider Vinegar
1 t	Sugar
-	Pepper and Garlic Salt to taste

In a large bowl, place mixed greens, shredded orange peel, and strawberries. Stir dressing and pour 3 Tablespoons Mandarin Orange Salad Dressing over salad. Sprinkle with pecans. Serves 1.

Blocked Salads
This salad can be eaten alone as a 3-block meal.

Grilled Chicken Salad with
Tomato-Basil Vinaigrette for 1

2-oz	Chicken Breast, skinless, boneless
1 C	Spinach, torn
3 C	Red-tip lettuce, torn
1	Sweet Pickle, small

Tomato-Basil
Vinaigrette
dressing:

1	Tomato, medium
2 t	Canola Oil
1 T	Red Wine Vinegar
1 t	Dried Basil, crushed
1 t	Sugar
1/4 t	Horseradish
1/8 t	Pepper
1	Garlic clove, minced

In a blender or food processor combine dressing ingredients. Cover and blend until smooth.
Grill Chicken and slice into thin strips. In a large mixing bowl, combine spinach, red-tip lettuce, and grilled chicken strips. Pour Tomato-Basil Vinaigrette over salad.

Blocked Salads
This salad can be eaten alone as a 3-block meal.

Fresh Fruit Salad with Grilled Chicken for 1
2 oz	Chicken Breasts: skinless, boneless
2 C	Red-tip lettuce, torn
1/4 C	Red Raspberries
1/4 C	Blackberries
1/4 C	Strawberries, halved

Lemon Yogurt Dressing:
2-oz	Vanilla Yogurt Custard
1/2 t	Canola Oil
1/2 T	Miracle Whip, regular
½ t	Lemon Peel, finely shredded

In small mixing bowl stir together dressing ingredients, cover and chill until ready to serve.
Combine lettuce, red raspberries, blackberries, and halved strawberries into each bowl. Pour dressing over the salad. Serves 1.

Blocked Salads
This salad can be eaten alone as a 3-block meal.

Grilled Chicken Salad with Raspberry Dressing for 1
2-oz	Chicken Breasts, skinless, boneless
10	Seedless Grapes, halved
1	Celery stalk, sliced
1 T	Pecan pieces
2 C	Red-tip Lettuce
1/4 C	Raspberries

Raspberry Dressing:
1/4 C	Raspberries
1 T	Sour Cream, fat free
2 T	Milk
1 t	Lemon Juice
1/8 t	Celery Seed

In a medium mixing bowl combine Lettuce, chopped grapes, celery, raspberries, and pecans. For dressing, in a screw-top jar, combine crush 1/4 C raspberries, sour cream, milk, lemon juice, and celery seed. Pour dressing over fruit mixture.

Blocked Salads
This salad can1 be eaten alone as a 3-block meal.

Grilled Chicken Salad with Avocado and Grapefruit for 1
2 oz	Chicken Breasts: skinless, boneless
2 C	Red-leaf Lettuce, torn
1/2	Grapefruit, medium peeled and sectioned
1/4	Avocado, medium, pitted, peeled, and sliced

Raspberry Vinaigrette Dressing:
1 t	Raspberry Vinegar
1/4 C	Raspberries
1 t	Sugar

Dressing:
Combine salad oil, raspberries and raspberry vinegar and pour in a screw-top jar. Cover and shake well.

Place lettuce in a salad bowl; arrange grapefruit sections and avocado slices, on the top. Shake dressing well and pour over salad. Makes 1 serving.

Blocked Salads
This salad can be eaten alone as a 3-block meal.

Ham Salad with Cranberry Vinaigrette for 1
2 oz	Diced Ham, 97% lean
3 C	Red-tip lettuce
1/2	Orange, medium, sectioned
3	Red Onion rings

Cranberry Vinaigrette:
2 T	Cranberry Juice Cocktail
1/2 T	Canola Oil
1 t	Cider Vinegar
1/8 t	Basil, dried, crushed
1/2 t	Sugar

Salad Dressing:
Combine all dressing ingredients, in a screw-top jar, cover and shake well.
In a large salad bowl, combine torn mixed greens, orange sections and red onions.
Shake Cranberry Vinaigrette well. Pour over salad. Toss lightly to coat.

Blocked Salads
This salad can be eaten alone as a 4-block meal.

Fresh Fruit Salad with Pecans and Grilled Chicken for 1
3 oz	Chicken Breasts: skinless, boneless
2 C	Red-tip lettuce, torn
1/2 C	Red Raspberries
1/2 C	Blackberries
1/2 C	Strawberries, halved
1/2 T	Pecans, chopped

Lemon Yogurt Dressing:
2 oz	Vanilla Yogurt Custard
1/2 t	Canola Oil
1/2 T	Miracle Whip
½ t	Lemon Peel, finely shredded

In a small mixing bowl Stir together dressing ingredients and place in a small mixing bowl. Cover and chill until ready to serve.

Grill chicken breasts and slice into thin strips.

Place lettuce the, red raspberries, blackberries, and strawberries into a bowl. Drizzle dressing over the top. Sprinkle on the pecans.

Blocked Salads
This salad can be eaten alone as a 3-block meal for 2 people.

Tropical Shrimp Salad with Fruit for 2
5	Lettuce Leaves
15	Shrimp, cooked and chilled
1/4	Avocado, sliced
1/2 C	Red Pepper, thin strips
1/2	Tomato, medium, diced

Apricot Preserve Dressing:
3 T	Sour Cream, fat free
3 T	Apricot preserves
1 T	Red Wine Vinegar
1/2 T	Canola Oil
1/2 T	Miracle Whip, fat free
1/2 T	Soy Sauce
1/2 t	Prepared Mustard
1/8 t	Ground Cinnamon

Stir together all the salad dressing ingredients. Cover and chill till ready to serve.

Line 2 plates with leaf lettuce. Arrange shrimp, avocado, pepper strips, and tomatoes on the lettuce-lined plates. Sprinkle with additional cinnamon, if desired. Pour dressing over salad.

Blocked Salads
This salad can be eaten alone as a 3-block meal for 3 people.

Overnight Vegetable Salad for 3

4 C	Mixed Greens, torn
1/2 C	Cauliflower flowerets
1/2 C	Broccoli flowerets
1 C	Cherry Tomatoes
1/2 C	Pea Pods
2	Sliced Radishes
1	Hard-boiled eggs, sliced
3 slices	Bacon, fried crisp, drain
3 T	Green onions: cut small
5 T	Miracle Whip, fat free
4 T	Sour Cream, fat free
2 T	Parmesan Cheese, fat free
2 T	Pesto Sauce
1-3 t	Milk 2%
2 oz	Cheddar Cheese, shredded, fat free

Place greens in the bottom of a 3-quart salad bowl. Layer in the following order: cauliflower, broccoli, cherry tomatoes, pea pods, radishes, hard-boiled eggs, bacon, and green onions.

Dressing:
Combine miracle whip, sour cream, Parmesan Cheese, and Pesto Sauce. If necessary, stir in milk to make dressing of desired consistency.

Spread dressing evenly over the top of the salad. Sprinkle with cheddar cheese. Cover tightly with plastic wrap. Chill for 4 to 24 hours. Toss lightly to mix. Makes 3 servings.

Blocked Salads
This salad can be eaten alone as a 4-block meal for 2 people.

Layered Tuna and Pasta Salad for 2

1 C	Macaroni (2 oz. dry)
2 C	Iceberg Lettuce, shredded
1/2 C	Tomato, chopped
4 oz	Tuna, albacore, water packed
1	Egg, hard boiled
2 T	Green Onions, sliced
1 oz	Cheddar Cheese, shredded, fat free

Herb Dressing:

4 T	Miracle Whip, fat free
2 T	Miracle Whip, regular
1/2 T	Lemon Juice
1/2 T	Dijon-style mustard
1/8 t	Black Pepper

Cook pasta according to package directions. Drain, rinse with cold water and drain again.

Place shredded lettuce in the bottom of a 3-quart salad bowl. Layer in the following order: cooked pasta, cucumber, tomato, tuna, peas, olives, egg slices, and green onions.

Carefully spread Herb Dressing evenly over top of salad, sealing to the edge of the bowl. Sprinkle with cheese. Cover tightly to mix. Makes 2 servings.

FOOD GUIDE SECTION

This section is to help you balance your own meals, or change the meals I have provided for you.

G/R stands for Glycemic Carbohydrate Rating. The Glycemic Rating rates how fast certain foods increase blood sugar levels, and how long it takes for you body to bring it back to normal.

The lower the Glycemic Rating numbers for the carbohydrates, the better your chances of losing weight faster, as they usually have more fiber, minerals and vitamins.

P stands for Protein grams, **C** is Carbohydrate grams, and **F** is Fat grams.

FOOD GUIDE SECTION

FOOD	SIZE	P	C	F
Beef, Raw				
Beef Brisket, extra lean	4 oz.	35.0	0	11.0
Beef Liver, baby	4 oz.	22.6	6.6	4.3
Beef Tenderloin	4 oz.	32.0	0	10.8
Bottom Round Steak, lean	12 oz.	80.2	0	12.8
Bottom Round Steak, lean	19 oz.	127.1	0	20.5
Canadian bacon, light, slices	2	5.5	0	0.7
Canadian bacon, Pizza Style, slices	22	9.0	0	4.0
Chuck, Arm Pot Roast, trimmed	3 oz.	28.1	0	6.5
Flank Steak, trimmed	3.5 oz.	27.0	0	10.0
Ground Beef, 93% lean	4 oz.	21.0	0	6.0
Ground Beef, 93% lean	15 oz.	78.7	0	22.5
Ground Beef, 93 % lean	16 oz.	84.0	0	24.0
Ground Sirloin, extra lean	4 oz.	30.0	0	9.0
Stew Beef, lean, (Bottom Round)	19 oz.	127.1	0	20.5
Round Steak, full cut	3 oz.	24.8	0	6.2
Round Tip, trimmed	3 oz.	24.4	0	5.0
Top Round, lean	4 oz.	30.7	0	4.3
Top Sirloin, lean	9 oz.	77.4	0	17.4
Chicken, Raw				
Breasts, Skinless	10.5 oz.	68.2	0	4.2
Breasts, Skinless	12 oz.	78.0	0	4.8
Drumstick, Skinless about 2 legs	4 oz.	23.2	0	4.0
Drumstick, Skinless about 6 legs	15 oz.	87.0	0	15.0
Thighs, Skinless	4 oz.	22.4	0	4.4
Lamb				
Leg, shank, lean	4 oz.	32.0	0	8.0
Sirloin, lean	4 oz.	32.0	0	10.0
Rack of Lamb	4 oz.	23.2	0	6.8
Pork, Raw				
Bacon, lean, slices	3	5.8	0.1	9.4
Breakfast Sausage, low fat (made with turkey and pork)	2	3.5	1.5	0.7
Ham, extra lean	5 oz.	30.0	0	8.0
Pork, Ground	1 oz.	4.8	0	6.0
Pork Loin Chops, lean ½" thick	4 oz.	24.8	0	8.0
Pork Tenderloin, trimmed, boneless	3 oz.	17.0	0	5.0
Teriyaki Tenderloin, Hormel	4 oz.	21.0	4.0	4.0
Anchovies, olive oil packed	6	4.0	0	1.5
Bass, Freshwater	6 oz.	28.0	0	0
Bass, Sea	5 oz.	33.0	0	4.0
Bass, Striped	5 oz.	30.0	0	4.0
Carp	6 oz.	30.0	0	10.0
Clams, raw	½ C	29.0	6.0	2.0
Cod, Atlantic	3 oz.	15.1	0	0.6
Crab, Alaskan King	6 oz.	32.0	0	1.0
Crabmeat, canned	4 oz.	30.0	0	2.0
Crayfish	5 oz.	33.0	0	2.0

FOOD GUIDE SECTION

FOOD	SIZE	P	C	F
Seafood, Raw				
Flounder	6 oz.	32.0	0	2.0
Haddock	6 oz.	28.0	0	0
Halibut	5 oz.	37.0	0	4.0
Lobster	6 oz.	32.0	0	2.0
Monkfish	6 oz.	31.0	0	3.0
Mussels	5 oz.	33.0	10.0	6.0
Orange Roughy	16 oz.	64.0	0	4.0
Oysters	1	5.0	3.0	1.0
Perch Ocean	6 oz.	36.9	0	3.6
Salmon; Coho	4 oz.	30.0	0	9.0
Salmon, Pink, 14¾ oz.	1 can	84.6	0	35.0
Salmon, smoked	6 oz.	31.0	0	9.0
Scallops	12 lg.	30.0	4.0	1.0
Shrimp, Steamed, lg.	12	25.7	0	1.7
Shrimp, Steamed	16 oz.	92.1	4.1	7.8
Shrimp, Salad Size	1C	14.0	2.0	2.0
Snapper	5 oz.	29.0	0	2.0
Sole	4 oz.	21.3	0	1.3
Swordfish	6 oz.	33.0	0	1.0
Rainbow Trout	6 oz.	34.0	0	6.0
Tuna, Albacore, water pack	4 oz.	30.0	0	2.0
Tuna, Blue Fin	5 oz.	33.0	0	7.0
Tuna, Yellow Fin	4 oz.	33.0	0	1.0
Turkey, Raw				
Breast, skinless	4 oz.	27.0	0	1.6
Breast, skinless	16 oz.	108.0	0	6.4
Breast, skinless, roasted	4 oz	34.0	0	1.0
Breast, skinless, ground	16 oz.	108.0	0	6.4
Dark meat, skinless	4 oz.	22.8	8	4.8
Dark Meat, skinless	16 oz.	91.2	0	19.2
Dark Meat, skinless, roasted	4 oz.	32.0	0	8.0
Dark meat, skinless	4 oz.	22.8	8	4.8
Veal				
Cutlets	3.5 oz.	26.3	0	4.2
Cutlets	10.5 oz.	79.0	0	18.4
Loin, skinless, roasted	4 oz.	29.0	0	8.0
Shoulder, skinless, roasted	4 oz.	29.0	0	7.0
Sirloin, skinless	3.5 oz.	20.0	0	3.1
Sirloin, skinless, roasted	4 oz.	30.0	0	7.0
Ground Veal	1 oz.	5.4	0	1.9
Venison				
Venison Burger	16 oz.	104.1	0	11.0
Venison, Raw	16 oz.	104.1	0	11.0
Venison, roasted	4 oz.	34.0	0	4.0

FOOD GUIDE SECTION

FOOD	SIZE	P	C	F
Lunch Meats				
Carl Buddig, 97%:				
Chicken Breast, oven roasted	2.5 oz.	13.0	1.0	1.0
Corn Beef, lean	2.5 oz.	14.0	0	5.0
Honey Ham, oven roasted	2.5 oz.	13.0	4.0	2.0
Pastrami, lean	2.5 oz.	14.0	1.0	5.0
Peppered Beef, lean	1 oz.	5.0	1.0	2.0
Smoked Turkey, lean	1 oz.	5.0	1.0	3.0
Turkey Breast, honey roasted, 99%	2.5 oz.	13.0	4.0	1.0
Cooked Ham, extra lean, 96% sliced	1	5.0	0	1.0
Healthy Choice, 97%:				
Chicken Breast, oven roast slices	1	6.0	1.0	0.9
Chicken Breast, deli-thin slices	1	10.0	0.9	0.9
Honey Ham, deli-thin slices	1	2.0	0.9	0.9
Turkey Breast	2 oz.	9.0	3.0	1.5
Turkey Breast, honey roasted	1 oz.	6.0	1.0	1.0
Turkey Breast, oven roasted	1 oz.	6.0	0.9	0.9
Healthy Deli:				
Corned Beef, lean	2 oz.	11.4	1.4	2.0
Hillshire Farm, 97% or 98%:				
Chicken Breast, smoked, deli-select	1 oz.	6.0	1.0	0.9
Corned Beef, 98%, deli-select	2 oz.	11.0	0	1.0
Honey Ham, 97%, deli select	2 oz.	10.0	2.0	1.5
Pastrami, 98%, deli-select	2 oz.	11.0	1.0	1.0
Roast Beef, 98%, deli-select	2 oz.	11.0	2.0	1.0
Louis Rich, 96%:				
Honey Ham, carving board	2.1 oz.	10.9	1.8	1.9
Turkey, oven roasted, white meat	1 oz.	4.9	0.1	1.7
Turkey Pastrami, deli-thin	1 oz.	2.0	0.9	0.9
Prosciutto	1 oz.	7.0	0	7.0
Nuts and Seeds Raw and Dry Roasted				
Almonds, slivered	1 T	3.0	3.0	8.0
Brazil Nuts, whole	6-8	4.0	3.0	18.8
Cashews, salted about 14 lg. or 26 sm.	1 oz.	5.0	8.0	13.0
Filberts/Hazelnuts	1 oz.	3.7	3.0	17.8
Peanuts, dry roasted	1 oz.	7.0	6.0	14.0
Peanuts, raw	1 T	4.0	3.0	7.0
Peanut Butter, Jif, (creamy or chunky)	1 T	4.0	5.0	8.0
Peanut Butter, other	1 T	4.0	3.0	7.0
Pecans, chopped	1 T	0.5	1.3	5.0
Pecans (about 10 whole med.)	1 oz.	2.0	5.0	19.0
Pine Nuts, raw	1 T	4.0	2.0	8.0
Pistachios, (about 47)	1 oz.	5.8	7.1	13.7

FOOD GUIDE SECTION

FOOD	SIZE	P	C	F
Nuts and Seeds Raw and Dry Roasted				
Pumpkin Seeds, roasted, about 85	1 oz.	5.3	6.0	5.5
Sesame Seeds	1 T	1.6	2.1	4.5
Soy Nuts	½ C	15.0	9.0	10.5
Spanish Peanuts	1 T	2.0	1.3	4.7
Sunflower Seeds, raw	1 T	3.0	3.0	8.0
Sunflower Seeds, dry roasted, salted	1 oz.	5.5	4.9	14.1
Walnuts, chopped raw	1 T	2.0	3.0	9.0
Walnuts, about 14 halves	1 oz.	4.0	3.0	17.6
Wheat Germ, original toasted	1 T	2.0	2.0	0.5
Dairy				
American Cheese, Healthy Choice	1	5.0	2.0	1.0
American Cheese, red. fat slices	1	4.0	2.0	3.0
American Cheese, fat-free slices	1	5.0	2.0	0
Blue Cheese Crumbles	1 oz	1.8	0.2	2.4
Brie, (Dorman's regular)	1 oz.	5.1	0.3	6.6
Camembert, (Dorman's 50 %)	1 oz.	5.6	0.3	7.3
Camembert, (Dorman's 45 %)	1 oz.	6.0	0.3	6.3
Cheddar Cheese, reg.	1 oz.	7.0	1.0	9.0
Cheddar Cheese, reg. Shredded	½ C	14.0	0.7	18.7
Cheddar Cheese, light	4 T	8.0	0.5	5.0
Cheddar Cheese, fat-free	1 oz.	8.0	1.0	0
Cool Whip, fat free	2 T	0	3.0	0
Cool Whip, fat free	¼ C	0	6.0	0
Cottage Cheese, 2 %	1 C	28.0	8.0	4.0
Cottage Cheese, 1 %	1 C	28.0	8.0	2.0
Cream Cheese, fat free	1 oz.	4.0	3.0	0
Cream Cheese, Philly light	1 T	1.5	1.0	2.5
Feta Cheese	1 oz.	4.0	1.2	6.0
Fiesta Blend Cheese, shredded	¼ C	6.0	0	9.0
Gouda Cheese (Kraft)	1 oz.	7.0	0	9.0
Gruyere Cheese	1 oz.	8.4	0.1	9.1
Havarti Cheese, regular	1 oz.	6.0	0	11.0
Havarti, (Dorman's) 60%	1 oz.	5.4	0.3	10.6
Havarti, (Dorman's) 45%	1 oz.	6.7	0.3	7.0
Milk, 2%	8 oz.	8.0	12.0	5.0
Milk, 1 %	8 oz.	8.0	12.0	3.0
Milk, skim	8 oz.	9.0	12.0	0
Milk, Nonfat Dry, mixed	1 C	8.0	12.0	0
Milk, Evaporated	½ C	8.6	12.6	9.5
Milk, Evaporated, skim	½ C	8.0	16.0	0
Monterey Jack, reg.	1 oz.	7.0	0.3	9.0
Monterey Jack, light	1 oz.	9.0	0.3	6.0
Mozzarella, Healthy Choice	¼ C	8.0	1.0	1.5
Mozzarella, reg., shredded	¼ C	7.0	0	6.0
Mozzarella, light	1 oz.	9.0	1.0	2.0

FOOD GUIDE SECTION

FOOD	SIZE	P	C	F
Dairy, continued				
Mozzarella, fat-free	1 oz.	9.0	0	0
Parmesan, grated, regular	1 T	3.0	0	2.3
Parmesan, grated, light	1 T	2.0	0.2	1.5
Parmesan, grated, fat free	1 T	1.5	4.5	0
Provolone, light	1 oz.	7.0	1.0	5.0
Ricotta, light	1 oz.	4.0	1.0	2.0
Sour Cream, light	1 T	1.0	1.0	1.0
Sour Cream, regular	1 T	0.4	0.5	2.5
Sour Cream, fat free	2 T	3.0	1.0	0
String Cheese, light	1 oz.	9.0	1.0	2.0
Swiss, light	1 oz.	8.0	1.0	6.0
Swiss, fat-free	1 oz.	8.0	1.0	0
Swiss, reg. slices	1	4.0	2.0	5.0
Swiss, fat free, slices	1	5.0	2.0	0
Velveeta. reg. about ¼" thick	1	4.0	2.0	6.0
Yogurt, plain, fat free	8 oz.	13.0	17.0	0
Yogurt, plain, light	8 oz.	12.0	16.0	3.0
Yoplait, light	6 oz.	6.0	13.0	0
Yoplait, Vanilla Custard Yogurt	4 oz.	5.0	20.0	3.0
Drinks and Mixes				
Balance 40-30-30 Strawberry, scoops	2	14.0	19.0	6.0
Balance 40-30-30 Strawberry, Milk 2%	8 oz.	22.0	31.0	11.0
Balance 40-30-30 Chocolate, scoops	2	14.0	20.0	6.0
Balance 40-30-30 Chocolate, Milk 2%	8 oz.	22.0	32.0	11.0
Balance 40-30-30 Vanilla, scoops	2	14.0	19.0	6.0
Balance 40-30-30 Vanilla, Milk 2%	8 oz.	22.0	31.0	11.0
Protein Powder	4 T	24.0	0	0
Whey Protein Powder	4 T	16.0	2.0	1.0
Fats and Oils				
Butter	1 T	0	0	11.0
Canola Oil	1 T	0	0	14.0
Cream Cheese, Philly light	1 T	1.5	1.0	2.5
Mayonnaise, regular	1 T	0	0	11.0
Mayonnaise, fat free	1 T	0	3.0	0
Mayonnaise, low-fat	1 T	0	1.0	5.0
Miracle Whip, regular	1 T	0	2.0	7.0
Miracle Whip, fat free	1 T	0	2.0	0
Olive Oil	1 T	0	0	14.0
Olives, green pitted, medium	5 med.	0	0	3.0
Olives, black, large	1	0	0.3	0.5
Olives, Greek style	5 med.	0	0	3.0
Oriental Sesame Oil	1 T	0	0	13.6
Safflower oil	1 T	0	0	14.0
Peanut Oil	1 T	0	0	14.0
Wheat Germ Oil	1 T	0	0	14.0

FOOD GUIDE SECTION

FOOD		SIZE	P	C	F
Eggs					
Egg Whole, large		1	6.0	0	5.0
Egg, White		1	4.0	0	0
Egg, Yolk		1	3.0	0	5.0
Egg substitute, liquid		½ C	15.0	0	4.0
Alcoholic Beverages					
Burgundy, Gallo		4 oz.	0	0.8	0
Cabernet Sauvignon, Gallo		4 oz.	0	0	0
Champagne, brut (Jacques Bonet)		4 oz.	0	2.1	0
Champagne, brut (Lejon)		4 oz.	0	3.4	0
Champagne, extra dry (Jacques Bonet)		4 oz.	0	3.4	0
Champagne, extra dry (Lejon)		4 oz.	0	2.1	0
Chaglis, Gallo		4 oz.	0	4.0	0
Chardonnay, Gallo		4 oz.	0	0	0
Chenin Blanc, Gallo		4 oz.	0	1.6	0
Marsala Wine		2 T	0	2.0	0
Rhine, Gallo		4 oz.	0	4.0	0
Reisling, Gallo, Johannisberg		4 oz.	0	1.6	0
Rose, Gallo Grenache		4 oz.	0	2.4	0
Rose, Gallo Red Rose		4 oz.	0	6.4	0
Rose, Gallo Vin Rose		4 oz.	0	2.8	0
Rye Whiskey, all proof		1 oz.	0	0	0
Scotch, all proof		1 oz.	0	0	0
Tequila, all proof		1 oz.	0	0	0
Vodka, all proof		1 oz.	0	0	0
Whiskey, all proof		1 oz.	0	0	0
Breads, and Starches					
Angel Food Cake Mix, 1/12	H	1	3.0	30.0	0
Bagel, Plain	H	1	8.0	38.0	1.0
Bagel, Raisin/Cinnamon	H	1	7.0	40.0	1.0
Biscuit, buttermilk	H	1	7.0	40.0	1.0
Bread Crumbs	H	½ C	7.0	39.0	3.0
Bread Crumbs, Bella	H	1 T	1.0	4.5	0.3
Bread Crumbs, Bella	H	¼ C	4.0	18.0	1.5
Bread Sticks, 7 5/8" long	H	1	1.0	7.0	1.0
Bread, Pumpernickel, Pepperidge Farm	H	1	3.0	11.8	1.0
Bread, Rye	H	1	2.0	11.0	1.0
Bread, Wheat, Home Made, slice	H	1	1.6	11.3	1.2
Bread, Wheat, Home Pride	H	1	2.0	14.0	1.0
Bread, Wheat, Pepperidge Farm, Light Style	H	1	2.0	7.0	0.5
Bread, White, Home Pride	H	1	1.0	14.0	1.0
Buns, Hamburger/Hot Dog	H	1	4.0	22.0	1.0
Buns, reduce calorie	H	1	4.0	18.0	1.0
Chinese Rice Noodles	H	½ C	3.0	15.0	5.0
Coco Wheats, (1/3 C dry)	H	1 C	3.3	24.0	1.3

FOOD GUIDE SECTION

FOOD	G/R	SIZE	P	C	F
Breads, and Starches, continued.					
Cornbread, slice	H	1	4.0	29.0	6.0
Cornbread Mix, Jiffy, dry	H	¼ C	2.0	27.0	4.0
Cornmeal, dry	H	¼ C	2.0	23.0	1.0
Cornstarch	H	1 T	0	7.0	0
Couscous, cooked	H	½ C	3.0	21.0	0
Crackers, Oyster	H	5	0	0.4	0
Crackers, Ritz, reg.	H	1	0.2	2.0	0.8
Crackers, Ritz, reg.	H	5	1.0	10.0	5.0
Crackers, Ry Krisp	H	7	3.0	18.0	5.0
Crackers, Saltine	H	1	0.2	2.0	0.4
Crackers, Saltine	H	5	1.0	10.0	2.0
Crackers, Waverly	H	1	0.2	2.0	0.7
Crackers, Waverly	H	5	1.0	10.0	3.5
Croissant	H	1	4.0	19.0	19.0
Croutons, plain	H	1 oz.	1.0	3.0	0
Croutons, seasoned	H	1 oz.	1.0	3.0	1.0
Dinner Rolls	H	1	3.0	15.0	1.0
Egg Noodles (2 oz. dry)	H	1 C	8.0	38.0	3.0
Egg Noodles, yolk free (2 oz. dry)	H	1¾ C	8.0	38.0	1.0
Egg White Powder, Just Whites		2 t	3.2	0	0
English Muffin	H	1	5.0	25.0	1.0
English Muffin, Toasting Bread	H	1	3.0	14.5	1.0
Fettucine	MH	1 oz.	4.0	20.0	1.0
Flour, White, all purpose	H	1 T	0.7	5.5	0
Flour, White, all-purpose	H	1 C	12.0	88.0	0
Flour, Whole Wheat	H	1 C	16.0	72.0	0
French Bread, 4.75 x 4"	H	1	4.0	26.0	2.0
Kaiser Rolls	H	1	2.8	14.9	1.2
Lasagna Noodles, cooked (2 oz dry)	MH	1 C	7.0	40.0	1.0
Linguine, cooked (2 oz dry)	MH	1 C	7.0	40.0	1.0
Macaroni, cooked (2 oz dry)	M	1 C	6.0	40.0	1.0
Milk & Egg Protein, heaping		2 T	21.0	2.0	1.5
Muffins, Bran	H	1	3.0	23.0	5.0
Muffins, Blueberry	H	1	3.0	27.0	4.0
Noodles, Chow Mein	H	1 C	3.8	24.0	13.2
Pancakes, 4" each	H	1	2.0	13.0	3.0
Pasta, cooked	M	1 C	12.0	56.0	2.0
Pasta Shells, medium, cooked	M	1 C	7.0	42.0	1.0
Pita Pocket, 6.5 diameter	H	1	6.0	35.0	2.0
Popcorn, Air Popped	VH	3 C	2.0	15.0	0
Potato, baked, large	VH	1	5.0	49.0	0
Potato, Mashed	VH	½ C	2.0	19.0	1.0
Potato, new red, small	VH	3	2.0	14.0	0
Pretzel Sticks	H	11	1.5	11.0	0.5
Rice, Brown, cooked (¼ C raw)	MH	1 C	3.0	34.0	2.0

FOOD GUIDE SECTION

FOOD	G/R	SIZE	P	C	F
Breads, and Starches, continued					
Rice, Wild, cooked (¼ C raw)	MH	1 C	6.0	33.0	0.5
Rice, White, cooked (¼ C raw)	MH	1 C	4.0	38.0	0
Spaghetti, Angel Hair, cooked (2 oz dry)	MH	2 oz.	7.0	38.0	1.0
Sweet Potato, each	MH	1	1.0	14.0	0
Stuffing, Stove Top, all flavors	H	½ C	4.0	20.2	9.0
Taco shell, medium	M	1	1.0	8.0	3.0
Tortilla, flour, 6" Manny	H	1	1.0	11.0	1.0
Wheat Bran		8 T	4.7	19.4	1.3
Wheat Germ, toasted		8 T	16.0	16.0	4.0
Cereals Cooked					
Coco Wheats, cooked (1/3 C dry)	H	1 C	3.3	24.0	1.3
Malt-O-Meal, cooked (3 T dry)	H	1 C	4.0	25.0	0
Oat Bran, cooked	H	½ C	3.0	12.0	1.0
Oatmeal, regular, cooked (1 C cooked)		½ C	5.0	23.0	3.0
Dry Cereals					
All Bran, Extra Fiber, Kellogg's		1 oz.	4.0	8.0	0
All Bran, Wheat Bran, Kellogg's		1 oz.	4.0	11.0	0.5
Bran Buds, Wheat Bran, Kellogg's		1 oz.	4.0	11.0	0.7
Bran Chex, Wheat & Corn, Kellogg's		1 oz.	2.9	18.0	0.8
Bran Flakes, Kellogg's		1 oz.	3.0	14.0	0
Cinnamon Toast Crunch, Post		1 oz.	1.0	21.0	3.0
Cinnamon Toast Crunch, General Mills		¾ C	1.0	23.0	3.5
Fiber One, General Mills		1 oz.	2.0	10.0	1.0
40% Bran Flakes, Kellogg's		1 oz.	3.6	18.0	0.5
Frosted Flakes, Kellogg's		1 oz.	1.0	25.0	0
Fruit 'N Nut Granola, Golden Temple		1 oz.	3.0	17.0	4.5
High Protein Granola, Golden Temple		1 oz.	4.0	17.0	3.5
Honey Almond Granola, Golden Temple		1 oz.	4.0	17.0	3.5
Honey Bunches of Oats almonds, Post		1 oz.	2.0	21.0	3.0
Honey Nut Toasted, Oatmeal Quaker		1 oz.	3.0	18.0	3.0
Honey Nut Cheerios, General Mills		1 oz.	3.1	21.5	0.7
Light Muesli, Golden Temple		1 oz.	3.0	18.0	1.0
Light 'N Crunchy Granola, G. Temple		1 oz.	4.0	17.0	4.5
Malt-O-Meal		3 T dry	4.0	26.0	0
Maple Almond Granola, Golden Temple		1 oz.	4.0	18.0	3.5
Most, Wheat Bran & Wheat		1 oz.	4.0	17.6	0.3
Multi-Bran Chex, Ralston		1 oz.	2.0	21.0	1.0
Natural Food Raisins Almond, G. Temple		1 oz.	3.0	20.0	1.0
Natural Oat & Wheat Germ, Heartland		1 oz.	2.9	17.7	4.4
Natural Food Raisins Almond, G. Temple		1 oz.	3.0	20.0	1.0
Natural Oat & Wheat Germ, Heartland		1 oz.	2.9	17.7	4.4
Oat Bran Almond, Golden Temple		1 oz.	4.0	17.0	3.5
Oat Bran Flakes, Arrowhead Mills		1 oz.	5.0	16.0	2.0
Oat Bran Granola, raisins & almonds		1 oz.	3.0	16.0	3.5
Oat Bran Flakes, Arrowhead Mills		1 oz.	5.0	16.0	2.0

FOOD GUIDE SECTION

FOOD	GR	SIZE	P	C	F
Dry Cereals, continued.					
Oat Bran Granola, raisins & almonds		1 oz.	3.0	16.0	3.5
Oat Bran Muesli, dates & almonds		1 oz.	3.0	19.0	1.5
Oat Bran Muesli, raisins & hazelnuts		1 oz.	3.0	17.0	1.5
Oat Flakes, Arrowhead Mills		1 oz.	1.0	15.5	4.0
Oat Flakes, Post		1 oz.	4.0	19.0	1.0
Oatbake Honey Bran, Kellogg's		1 oz.	2.0	18.0	3.0
Oatbake Raisin Nut, Kellogg's		1 oz.	2.0	18.0	3.0
Oatmeal Crisp, General Mills		1 oz.	3.0	20.0	2.0
100% Bran, wheat bran & barley, Nabisco		1 oz.	3.5	19.0	1.4
100% Natural Almond, Golden Temple		1 oz.	3.0	16.0	4.0
100% Natural mixed grain, Quaker		1 oz.	3.0	16.0	5.5
100% Natural mixed grain, raisins		1 oz.	3.0	19.0	2.0
100% Natural Oat Bran, Golden Temple		1 oz.	5.0	14.0	2.5
Raisin Bran Wheat, Kellogg's		1.3 oz.	4.0	24.0	0.7
Raisin Bran Wheat, Post		1 oz.	2.6	17.5	0.5
Shredded Wheat, biscuit, Nabisco		1	2.0	16.0	1.0
Special K, Kellogg's		1 oz.	5.6	20.6	0.1
Total Wheat, General Mills		1 oz.	2.8	19.0	0.6
Wheat Chex, Ralston		1 oz.	2.8	23.0	0.7
Wheaties, General Mills		1 oz.	2.7	22.0	0.5
Sauces & Broths					
Alfredo Sauce		¼ C	6.5	3.0	15.0
Béarnaise Sauce		2 T	0.5	0.2	21.0
Cider Vinegar		1 T	0	0.9	0
Cocktail Sauce, Marzetti		¼ C	1.0	12.0	0.5
Cream Sauce		¼ C	0.5	0.7	25.0
Marinara Sauce		½ C	4.0	9.0	5.0
Mustard, French's		1 T	0	0	0
Mustard, Grey Poupon		1 T	0	0	0
Soy Sauce		1 T	1.0	1.0	0
Tomato Sauce		15 oz.	7.0	21.0	0
Worcestershire Sauce		1 T	0	0	0
SoupsChunky, Campbell's					
Turkey Vegetable		1 Can	9.0	16.0	6.0
Old Fashioned Vegetable Beef		1 Can	13.0	20.0	6.0
Soups, Campbell's condensed					
Beef with Vegetables & Barley		1 Can	12.5	27.5	5.0
Cheddar Cheese		1 Can	5.2	13.1	7.8
Chicken Noodle		1 Can	7.5	20.0	5.0
Chicken with Wild Rice		1 Can	7.5	20.0	5.0
Minestrone		1 Can	5.2	13.6	3.0
Tomato, unprepared		1 Can	5.0	39.1	4.7
Vegetarian Vegetable		1 Can	7.5	40.0	2.5

FOOD GUIDE SECTION

FOOD	G/R	SIZE	P	C	F
Soups, Campbell's, Home Cookin'					
Chicken Minestrone		1 Can	15.0	9.0	6.0
Chicken Rice		1 Can	12.0	9.0	5.0
Soups, Campbell's, Ready to Serve					
Chicken With Rice		1 Can	10.0	16.0	4.0
Chunky Beef		1 Can	15.0	24.0	5.0
Chunky Chicken Noodle		1 Can	14.0	20.0	7.0
Soups, Mix					
Chicken Noodle, in broth Lipton's		1 Pkg.	8.0	36.0	8.0
Onion Soup, Lipton's, + 16 oz. sour cream fat free		1 Pkg.	24.0	24.0	0
Fruits and Juices, fresh and frozen					
Apple medium, whole	M	1	0	17.5	0
Apple Juice, Musselman's	M	4 oz.	0	15.0	0
Applesauce, Musselman's unsweetened	M	½ C	0	14.0	0
Applesauce, Musselman's, regular	M	½ C	0	20.0	0
Apricots	MH	3	1.0	12.0	0
Apricots, light syrup	MH	½ C	0.7	15.4	0.4
Apricots, in juice	MH	½ C	0	17.0	0
Avocado	L	¼	1.0	3.0	8.0
Banana	H	1	1.0	25.0	1.0
Blackberries	L	½ C	0.5	5.6	0
Blackberries, frozen, light syrup	L	½ C	0.9	24.0	0.3
Blueberries	L	½ C	1.0	10.0	0
Cantaloupe	L	½	2.0	20.0	0
Cantaloupe, cubed	L	1 C	1.4	13.4	0.4
Cherries, sweet	L	½ C	1.0	10.0	1.0
Cranberry Juice Cocktail, Ocean Spray	L	8 oz.	0.5	26.0	0
Cranberry Sauce	H	¼ C	0	27.0	0
Cranberry Sauce, Whole Berry	H	¼ C	0	11.0	0
Fruit Cocktail, light	L	½ C	0	14.0	0
Grapefruit, White, 3¾" diameter	L	½	1.0	10.0	0
Grapefruit, Pink & Red, 3¾" diameter	L	½	0.6	11.9	0
Grapefruit, canned, in Juice	L	½ C	0	9.0	0
Grapefruit, canned, light syrup	L	½ C	0	20.0	0
Grapefruit Juice, Ocean Spray	L	6 oz.	1.0	16.0	0
Grapefruit Juice, pink, Ocean Spray	L	6 oz.	1.0	15.0	0
Grapefruit Juice, Red, Ocean Spray	L	6 oz.	1.0	14.0	0
Grapes	M	10	0	5.0	0
Guava, cubed	M	½ C	1.0	14.0	1.0
Honeydew Melon, cubed	L	1 C	0.8	14.6	0
Kiwi Fruit, medium	L	1	1.0	11.0	0
Lemon or Lime juice	M	1 T	0	1.0	0
Mango, cubed	MH	½ C	1.0	14.0	0

FOOD GUIDE SECTION

FOOD	G/R	SIZE	P	C	F
Fruits and Juices, fresh and frozen, continued.					
Mandarin Oranges, light canned	M	½ C	1.0	16.0	0
Nectarine, medium	M	1	1.0	14.0	0
Orange, medium	M	1	1.0	12.5	0
Orange Juice, frozen	M	¼ C	0.6	63.3	0
Orange Juice, Tropicana	M	3 oz.	0.6	9.75	0
Orange Juice, Tropicana	M	4 oz.	0.8	13.0	0
Papaya, cubed	H	½ C	0	11.0	0
Peach, fresh, 2 ½"	L	1	0	9.0	0
Peach, fresh, sliced	L	½ C	0.6	8.1	0
Peach, canned, light, sliced	L	½ C	0	22.0	0
Peach, canned, in Juice	L	½ C	0	14.0	0
Peach, slices, frozen, sweetened	L	½ C	0.8	29.0	0
Pear, fresh, 2 ½" diameter	L	1	0	21.0	0
Pear, light syrup	L	½ C	0.2	19.0	0
Pear, in juice	L	½ C	0.4	15.0	0
Pineapple, fresh	L	1 C	1.0	17.5	0
Pineapple, light syrup	L	½ C	0.5	16.0	0
Pineapple, in juice	L	½ C	0.5	17.0	0
Plum, medium	L	1	0.5	8.0	0
Plum, light syrup	L	½ C	0.5	20.5	0
Plum, juice	L	½ C	0.7	19.1	0
Prunes, pitted	M	2	0	11.0	0
Raisins, dark, seedless, packed	H	½ C	3.0	61.0	0
Raisins, golden, seedless, packed	H	½ C	3.0	63.0	0
Raspberries, Red, Black, Yellow	L	1 C	0	6.0	0
Raspberries, frozen, light syrup	L	½ C	0.8	20.0	0.8
Strawberries	L	1 C	1.0	7.0	0
Strawberries, frozen, unsweetened	L	½ C	0.5	10.4	0.1
Strawberries, frozen, light syrup	L	½ C	0.6	22.0	0
Sunny Delight	M	2 oz.	0	7.25	0
Sunny Delight	M	3 oz.	0	10.8	0
Tangerine	M	1	0	9.0	0
Watermelon, diced	M	1 C	1.0	11.0	0
Jams/Jellies					
Este, all flavors		1 t	0	0	0
Featherweight, all flavors		1 t	0	1.0	0
Homemade, Light, all flavors 1 t			0	3.0	0
Kraft, all flavors		1 t	0	4.0	0
Smucker's Slenderella, all flavors		1 t	0	2.0	0
Preserves					
Apple Butter		1 t	0	3.0	0
Knott's Berry Farm, all flavors		1 t	0	4.0	0
Polaner, all flavors		1 t	0	4.5	0

FOOD GUIDE SECTION

FOOD	G/R	SIZE	P	C	F
Vegetables, canned					
Anchovies, olive oil packed		6	4.0	0	1.5
Asparagus Spears		15 oz.	7.0	7.0	0
Beets, cut		15 oz.	3.0	21.0	0
Corn		½ C	3.0	20.0	1.0
Enchilada Sauce, Old El Paso		10 oz.	0	13.5	3.5
French Fried Onion, canned		2 T	0	3.0	3.5
Garbanzo Beans, canned		½ C	5.0	16.0	1.0
Green Beans		1 C	2.0	8.0	0
Green Chiles, diced		4 oz.	0	4.0	0
Hormel Chili w/o beans		1 C	15.0	14.0	9.0
Jalapenos, sliced		¼ C	0	2.0	0
Kidney Beans		15½ oz.	28.0	4.9	0
Lima Beans		½ C	0.6	17.5	0.5
Mushrooms		4 oz.	1.0	2.0	0
Peas, Green		½ C	4.0	9.0	0
Pickles, Sweet, small		2	0	8.0	0
Pickle Relish, Sweet		1 T	0	4.0	0
Pickle, Dill, med.		1	0	1.0	0
Pimeinto		2 oz.	0.6	2.6	0.2
Pinto Beans		½ C	8.0	11.0	1.0
Pizza Sauce, Contadina		15 oz.	7.0	21.0	3.5
Refried Beans, fat free		½ C	8.0	14.0	0
Tomato Paste		2 T	1.0	5.0	0
Tomato Paste		6 oz.	5.0	25.0	0
Tomato Sauce		15 oz.	7.0	14.0	0
Sauerkraut		2 T	0	1.0	0
Sauerkraut		14.5 oz.	0	14.0	0
Stewed Tomatoes, Italian Recipe		14.5 oz.	3.5	17.5	0
Sweet Potatoes, candied		½ C	1.0	60.0	0
Whole Tomatoes		28 oz.	7.0	21.0	0
Yams		½ C	1.0	28.0	0
Vegetables, fresh					
Alfalfa sprouts	L	1 C	1.0	1.0	0
Artichoke, cooked, medium	L	1	4.0	14.0	0
Artichokes, canned	L	4 oz.	3.9	11.4	0.2
Asparagus, raw spears	L	5	2.0	0	0
Avocado	L	¼	1.0	3.0	8.0
Avocado, California, pureed	L	½ C	2.4	8.0	19.9
Avocado, Florida, pureed	L	½ C	1.8	10.3	10.2
Baked Beans, B&M	MH	1 C	15.0	48.0	6.0
Baked Beans, Van Camp	MH	1 C	11.0	52.0	2.0
Bamboo shoots	L	½ C	2.0	4.0	0
Bean Sprouts	L	½ C	4.0	7.0	0
Black Beans	M	½ C	8.0	20.0	1.0
Bok Choy	L	½ C	0	1.0	0

FOOD GUIDE SECTION

FOOD	G/R	SIZE	P	C	F
Vegetables, fresh, continued					
Broccoli, raw	L	1 C	3.0	6.0	0.5
Butternut Squash	M	½ C	1.0	11.0	0
Brussels Sprouts, raw	L	1 C	6.0	20.0	1.0
Cabbage, shredded, raw	L	1 C	1.0	4.0	0
Carrots, raw	H	1 C	2.0	23.0	0
Cauliflower	L	1 C	2.0	5.0	0
Cilantro, fresh	L	¼ C	0.1	0.1	0.1
Chili Pepper	L	¼ C	0	2.0	0
Celery stalk, raw, diced	L	1	0	2.0	0
Corn, frozen	H	½ C	2.0	14.0	1.0
Corn on the cob, ear	H	1	4.0	28.0	1.0
Cucumber, sliced	L	½ C	0	1.0	0
Eggplant, cubed	L	1 C	1.0	7.0	0
Endive, raw	L	½ C	0	1.0	0
Garlic Clove	L	1 T	0	0	0
Garlic powder	L	1 t	0	0	0
Ginger, fresh	L	1 t	0	0	0
Ginger powder	L	1 T	0	0	0
Green Beans, fresh	M	½ C	1.0	2.7	0.1
Green Onions, diced	L	¼ C	0.5	1.2	0
Green Pepper, diced	L	½ C	0.4	5.6	0.1
Hummus	L	¼ C	3.0	13.0	6.0
Jicama (Chinese Yam, Mexican Potato)	H	½ C	0.8	5.0	0.1
Kale, boiled	L	½ C	1.0	4.0	0
Leeks, raw	L	¼ C	1.0	4.0	0
Lentils, boiled	M	½ C	9.0	20.0	0
Lettuce, Iceberg	L	1 C	2.0	5.0	0
Lettuce, Butter head, leaves	L	5	0	1.0	0
Lettuce, Romaine	L	1 C	3.0	5.0	0
Lima Beans	M	½ C	7.0	20.0	0
Navy Beans, boiled	M	½ C	8.0	24.0	1.0
Mushrooms, raw	L	½ C	1.0	1.1	0.2
Mustard Greens	L	½ C	1.0	1.0	0
Okra, boiled	L	½ C	1.0	6.0	0
Onions, raw, chopped	L	½ C	0.9	5.6	0.1
Parsley, chopped	L	1 T	0	1.0	0
Peas, frozen	L	½ C	3.7	6.0	0.2
Pickles, dill	L	1	0	3.0	0
Pickles, sweet medium	H	1	0	8.0	0
Poi	H	½ C	1.0	33.0	0
Potatoes, Baked, large	VH	1	5.0	49.0	0
Potatoes, Mashed	VH	½ C	2.0	19.0	1.0
Potatoes, New Red, small	VH	3	2.0	14.0	0
Radishes, Red	L	4	0	1.0	0
Salsa, Pace	L	2 T	0	3.0	0
Sauerkraut	L	½ C	0	4.0	0

FOOD GUIDE SECTION

FOOD	G/R	SIZE	P	C	F
Vegetables, fresh, continued					
Snow Peas, raw	L	½ C	2.0	6.0	0
Spinach, raw	L	1 C	2.0	2.0	0
Summer Squash, boiled	M	½ C	1.0	4.0	0
Swiss Chard, raw, chopped	L	½ C	1.6	0.4	0
Sweet Potatoes, raw, cubes	VH	½ C	1.1	14.0	0.2
Swiss Chard, raw	L	½ C	0	1.0	0
Tempeh	L	½ C	0	1.0	0
Tofu, extra-firm	L	4 oz.	12.0	1.0	6.0
Tofu, soft	L	4 oz.	8.0	2.0	5.0
Tomato, medium	L	1	1.0	6.0	0
Tomato, raw, chopped	L	½ C	0	3.0	0
Turnips, boiled	L	½ C	1.0	6.0	0
Turnip Greens	L	½ C	1.0	3.0	0
Watercress		½ C	0.4	0	0
Yams, cubed, raw	MH	½ C	1.1	17.8	0.1
Zucchini, raw	L	½ C	1.0	2.0	0
Miscellaneous					
Betagen (EAS)		1½ t	0	2.0	0
Cocoa, Powder, sugar free		1 T	1.0	2.0	0.5
Honey		1 T	0	17.0	0
Molasses, light, mild		1 T	0	15.0	0
Myoplex (EAS)		2 oz.	25.0	20.0	1.5
Brown Sugar		1 T	0	12.0	0
White Sugar		1 T	0	12.0	0
Yeast		4½ T	6.9	1.9	0.7
40-30-30 Balance Bars					
Almond Brownie, 1 block		½ bar	7.0	10.0	3.0
Almond Brownie, 2 blocks		1 bar	14.0	20.0	6.0
Almond Butter Crunch, 1-block		½ bar	7.0	9.5	3.5
Almond Butter Crunch, 2-blocks1 bar			14.0	19.0	7.0
Banana Coconut, 1-block		½ bar	7.0	10.0	3.0
Banana Coconut, 2-blocks		1 bar	14.0	20.0	6.0
Carmel Nut Blast, 2-blocks		1 bar	15.0	22.0	7.0
Chocolate, 1-block		½ bar	7.0	10.5	3.0
Chocolate, 2-blocks		1 bar	14.0	21.0	6.0
Chocolate Raspberry Fudge, 1 block		½ bar	7.0	10.5	3.0
Chocolate Raspberry Fudge, 2 blocks		1 bar	14.0	21.0	6.0
Cranberry, 1 block		½ bar	7.0	9.0	3.0
Cranberry, 2-blocks		1 bar	14.0	18.0	6.0
Honey Peanut, 1 block		½ bar	7.0	10.5	3.0
Honey Peanut, 2 blocks		1 bar	14.0	21.0	6.0
Toasted Crunch, 1 block		½ bar	7.5	10.0	3.0
Toasted Crunch, 2-blocks		1 bar	15.0	20.0	6.0
Yogurt Honey Peanut, 1-block		½ bar	7.0	10.5	3.0
Yogurt Honey Peanut, 2 blocks		1 bar	14.0	21.0	6.0

FOOD GUIDE SECTION

FOOD	GR	SIZE	P	C	F
Snacks					
Doritos Nacho Cheesiest (about 11)		1 oz.	2.0	16.0	7.0
Doritos Nacho Spicy (about 12)		1 oz.	2.0	17.0	1.0
Fruit Gushers pouch		1	0	20.0	1.0
Gardetto's Snack-ems (about 34)		½ C	3.0	17.0	9.0
Jello Chocolate Pudding, prepared 2% Milk		1 C	5.0	13.0	3.0
M&M Mini's		3 oz.	6.0	54.0	21.0
Pringles Sour Cream & Onion Potato Chips (14)		1 oz.	2.0	14.0	10.0
Ruffles Chips (about 12)		1 oz.	2.0	13.0	10.0
Wow Original Chips (about 17)		1 oz.	2.0	17.0	0
Pringles, Fat Free, Potato Chips, Original (15)		1 oz.	2.0	15.0	0
Salad Dressing, bottled & home made					
Balsamic Vinaigrette, Girard's fat free		2 T	0	6.0	0
Balsamic Vinaigrette, Newmans		2 T	0	3.0	9.0
Barbecue Sauce, Open Pit		2 T	0	11.0	0.5
Barbecue Sauce, Open Pit		1 C	0	88.0	4.0
Chi-Chi's Seasoning Mix		7 t	0	7.0	0
Cocktail Sauce		¼ C	1.0	12.0	0.5
Heinz 57 Steak Sauce		1 T	0	4.0	0
Ketchup, Heinz		1 T	0	4.0	0
Mustard, French's		1 T	0	0	0
Old El Paso Taco Seasoning Mix		1 pkg.	0	30.0	0
Ortega Fajita Mix		1½ t	0	3.0	0
Slaw Dressing, light (Marzetti)		2 T	0	10.0	7.0
Mandarin Orange Salad Dressing, home made		2 T	0	0.4	2.3
Stir Fry Sauce (93% FF)		1 T	0	3.0	1.0
Sweet Pickle Relish		1 T	0.1	5.3	0.1
Thousand Island Dressing, regular		2 T	0	5.0	10.0
Thousand Island Dressing, fat free		2 T	0	8.0	0
Teriyaki Marinade, home made		15 T	6.0	11.5	14.0
White Sauce, home made		½ C	4.0	7.8	2.5

Index

Index

Breakfast	Blocks	Page
Cinnamon Toast Crunch	3	137
Cottage Cheese and Blackberries	2	130
Cottage Cheese and Canned Peaches	2	129
Cottage Cheese and Crushed Pineapple	2	129
Cottage Cheese and Fresh Peaches	2	129
Cottage Cheese and Fruit Cocktail	2	129
Cottage Cheese and Mandarin Oranges	2	129
Cottage Cheese and Raspberries	2	130
Cottage Cheese and Strawberries	2	130
Egg with Cheese and Strawberries	2	132
Egg with Cheese	2	132
Eggs and Ham with English Toasting Bread	4	143
Eggs and Cheese with English Toasting Bread	3	133
Eggs and Grapefruit	2	131
Eggs and Salsa	3	141
Eggs and Sausage with Potatoes and Jam	3	135
Eggs and Sausage with Potatoes and Strawberries	3	135
Eggs Benedict	3	135
Eggs with Cheese and Bacon	3	134
Eggs with Ham and Cheese	3	134
Eggs with Ham and Orange Juice	3	137
Eggs with Ham and Salsa	3	134
Eggs with Potatoes and Sausage	3	136
Eggs with Toast and Ham	4	142
Eggs with Toast and Jam	3	133
French Toast with Ham	3	136
French Toast with Ham and Orange Juice	4	142
French Toast with Sausage	4	143
Frosted Flakes	3	139
Ham and Eggs with Grapefruit	3	140
Ham and Eggs with Salsa and English Toasting Bread	4	142
Ham and Eggs with Toast and Sausage	4	140
Ham and Eggs with Toast and Strawberries	4	140
Honey Bunches of Oats with Almonds	3	138
Malt-O-Meal	3	141
Nutritionally Balanced Bar	2	131
Nutritionally Balanced Shake	2	132
Oatmeal	3	138
Omelet with Ham and Cheese	3	133
Omelet with Ham and Orange Juice	4	142
Omelet with Ham and Salsa	3	136
Poached Egg with Cantaloupe	2	131
Poached Egg with English Toasting Bread	2	130
Sausage and Egg with Orange Juice	3	132
Sausage and Eggs with Cantaloupe	3	139
Shredded Wheat	3	137
Smart Start	3	139
Special K	3	137
Tortilla	3	133
Wheat Chex	3	138
Wheaties	3	137

Index

Lunch	Blocks	Page
Beef with Vegetable and Barley and Tuna Sandwich	3	152
Beef with Vegetable and Barley Soup	2	147
BLT with American Cheese	2	148
BLT with Cheese	3	149
Chicken Noodle and Turkey Salad Sandwich	4	153
Chicken Noodle Soup and Ham Sandwich	3	150
Chicken Noodle Soup with Chips	2	148
Chicken Noodle Soup	2	147
Chicken with Wild Rice Soup	2	147
Chunky Beef Soup, Ready to Serve	3	152
Egg Salad Sandwich	2	148
Grilled Ham and Cheese Sandwich	2	146
Grilled Parmesan Beef Burger	4	155
Grilled Parmesan Turkey Burger	4	155
Ham and American Cheese Sandwich with Grapes	3	150
Ham and American Cheese Sandwich with Tangerine	3	151
Ham and American Cheese Sandwich	3	149
Ham and Swiss Cheese Sandwich 1½	4	153
Ham and Swiss Cheese Sandwich	3	150
Ham Sandwich 1½ with Grapes	4	154
Ham Sandwich 1½ with Tangerine	4	154
Hot Ham and Swiss	3	149
Hot Pastrami	3	152
Minestrone Soup	2	148
Patty Melt with Ground Beef and Smothered Onions	4	154
Patty Melt with Ground Turkey and Smothered Onions	4	156
Reuben Sandwich	4	156
Roast Beef Sandwich	3	149
Southwestern Cheeseburger	4	155
Tavern Hamburger	2	146
Toasted Tomato Sandwich with Cottage Cheese 2%	2	147
Tuna Melt	3	151
Tuna Sandwich	3	151
Turkey Salad Sandwich	2	146
Vegetarian Vegetable Soup and Grilled Ham and Cheese	4	153
Vegetarian Vegetable Soup and Ham Sandwich	3	152
Vegetarian Vegetable Soup	2	147

Index

Beef Dinner .... **Blocks** .... **Page**

- Beef Bourguignon for 4 .... 4 178
- Beef Burrito's for 3 .... 4 167
- Beef Fajita's for 3 .... 4 168
- Beef Liver Smothered in Onions 4 179
- Beef Stew for 4 .... 5 161
- Beef Stroganoff for 3 .... 5 159
- Beef Top Round with Horseradish Sauce for 3 .... 4 164
- Beef Top Round with Vegetables for 3 .... 4 165
- Bottom Round Roast and Vegetables for 3 .... 5 176
- Braised Beef with Vegetables and Barley for 3 .... 4 158
- Lasagna for 6 .... 5 171
- Meat Loaf for 3 .... 4 160
- Minnesota Taco's for 3 .... 5 169
- Moussaka for 3 .... 3 177
- Pepper Steak Stir Fry for 3 .... 4 163
- Roast Beef with Vegetables for 6 .... 4 180
- Shredded Beef Chimichangas for 3 .... 4 166
- Spaghetti for 6 .... 4 162
- Steak and Fries for 3 .... 4 175
- Steak and Potatoes for 3 .... 4 172
- Texas Hash for 4 .... 4 170
- Veal Scaloppini for 3 .... 5 173
- Veal with Vegetables and Gravy for 3 .... 4 174

Index

Chicken Dinner .... Blocks .... Page

    Chicken a la Marengo for 3 .... 4 194
    Chicken and Artichokes for 3 .... 4 188
    Chicken and Stuffing Bake for 3 .... 4 199
    Chicken Breasts with Sour Cherry Sauce for 3 .... 4 185
    Chicken Bruschetta for 3 .... 4 204
    Chicken Cacciatore for 3 .... 4 193
    Chicken Cordon Bleu for 3 .... 5 202
    Chicken Cutlet Parmesan for 3 .... 4 187
    Chicken Diane for 3 .... 4 203
    Chicken Dijon with Ginger Pear Sauce for 3 .... 4 207
    Chicken Drumsticks with Angel Food Cake for 3 .... 5 198
    Chicken Drumsticks with Salad for 3 .... 5 197
    Chicken Stir Fry for 3 .... 4 205
    Chicken Thighs with Sour Cherry Sauce for 3 .... 4 186
    Chicken with Orange Peel Szechwan for 3 .... 4 190
    Chicken with Peach Sauté for 3 .... 4 191
    Coq au Vin Blanc (Chicken with White Wine) for 3 .... 4 210
    Cranberry Chicken for 3 .... 4 183
    Garlic Chicken with Angel Food Cake for 3 .... 4 196
    Garlic Chicken with Ham Salad for 3 .... 4 195
    Grilled Chicken Vegetable Packet for 3 .... 4 209
    Hawaiian Chicken for 3 .... 4 192
    Honey Orange Chicken Stir Fry for 3 .... 4 184
    Manhattan Chicken for 3 .... 4 189
    Mushroom Garlic Chicken with Artichokes for 3 .... 4 206
    Orange Chicken with Green Grapes for 3 .... 4 208
    Oriental Chicken for 3 .... 5 182
    Sesame Chicken 211
    Teriyaki Chicken with Cole Slaw for 3 .... 4 200
    Teriyaki Chicken with Fruit Salad for 3 .... 4 201

Index

Fish Dinners	Blocks	Page
Baked Salmon Fillets with Apple Glaze for 3	4	214
Cheesy Fish Fillet for 3	4	229
Cheesy Orange Roughy for 3	4	224
Fillet of Sole for 3	4	226
Fish and Chips for 3	4	220
Grilled Halibut for 3	4	232
Grilled Orange Roughy with Apple Cole Slaw for 3	4	228
Grilled Salmon Fillets with Wild Rice for 3	4	213
Grilled Salmon with Blue Cheese Crumbles	5	219
Grilled Salmon with Lemon Dill Mayonnaise	5	218
Grilled Salmon with Lemon Rosemary Marinade	4	215
Grilled Swordfish with Mustard Sauce	4	216
Grilled Tuna Steak with Ginger Lime Marinade	4	217
Marinated Shrimp in Almond Sauce for 3	4	231
Orange Roughy for 3	4	230
Oriental Stir Fry Shrimp for 3	4	227
Salmon Patties for 3	5	222
Shrimp Scampi for 3	4	221
Stuffed Orange Roughy for 3	4	225

Pork Dinners	Blocks	Page
Boneless B.B.Q. Ribs for 3	4	234
Baked Pork Loin Chops with Sweet Potatoes for 3	4	233
Pork Chops with Stuffing for 3	4	236
Pork Loin Chops with Cole Slaw for 3	4	235
Pork Roast and Vegetables for 3	5	239
Pork Teriyaki with Chocolate Mousse for 3	5	238
Pork Teriyaki with Mandarin Orange Salad for 3	4	237

Vegetarian Dinner Choices	Blocks	Page
Eggplant Parmesana for 3	4	241
Spicy Vegetarian Lasagna	6	242
Vegetarian Chili	3	243
Vegetarian Fried Rice	3	244

Miscellaneous	Blocks	Page
2-Block Snacks		247
Balanced 3-Block Salads		263
Beef Dinners		158
Chicken Dinners		182
Fish Dinners		213
Pork Dinners		233
Holiday Section		253
Miscellaneous Choices		256
Salad Dressings, Marinades and Sauces		259

References

Art Ulene, Dr. "Book of Food Counts," Avery Publishing Group, 1996

Daoust, Joyce and Gene, "40-30-30 Fat Burning Nutrition," Wharton Publishing, 1995

Sears, Barry, Ph.D. "The Zone." Regan Books, Harper Collins Publishing, 1995

Sears, Barry, Ph.D. "Mastering the Zone," Regan Books, Harper Collins Publishing, 1997

Nutritional Guides from Fast Food Restaurants

About the Author

A homemaker for 40 years, I enjoy cooking for family and friends. Having grown up on a farm, I enjoy traditional "Down Home" recipes. When I discovered the Zone Diet, I struggled to balance those old recipes and subsequently developed a recipe collection of meals that are very flavorful and satisfying, and at the same time allow you to lose weight dramatically and healthfully.

Printed in the United States
25578LVS00003B/7-8